W9-BWP-935

# EMBARRASSMENT

# EMOTIONS AND SOCIAL BEHAVIOR

*Series Editor*
**Peter Salovey,** *Yale University*

Embarrassment: Poise and Peril in Everyday Life
*Rowland S. Miller*

Social Anxiety
*Mark R. Leary and Robin M. Kowalski*

Breaking Hearts: The Two Sides of Unrequited Love
*Roy F. Baumeister and Sara R. Wotman*

Jealousy: Theory, Research, and Clinical Strategies
*Gregory L. White and Paul E. Mullen*

# EMBARRASSMENT
## Poise and Peril in Everyday Life

ROWLAND S. MILLER

THE GUILFORD PRESS
New York   London

©1996 The Guilford Press
A Division of Guilford Publications, Inc.
72 Spring Street, New York, NY 10012

Last digit is print number:  9  8  7  6  5  4  3  2  1

**Library of Congress Cataloging-in-Publication Data**

Miller, Rowland S.
  Embarrassment : poise and peril in everyday life / Rowland S. Miller
      p.     cm. — (Emotions and social behavior)
  Includes bibliographical references and index.
  ISBN  1–57230–127–9
  1. Embarrassment.  I. Title.  II. Series.
BF575.E53M55  1996
152.4—dc20                                                        96–21200
                                                                         CIP

*To Jon, Chris, and Gale*

# Acknowledgments

~

I am grateful for the invaluable support and counsel of Mark Leary, who read the entire manuscript and provided constructive feedback. As you'll see, Mark figures prominently in this book due to the enormous quality (and quantity) of his own work on impression management and social anxiety. Series Editor Peter Salovey was also a thoughtful, compassionate critic; his advice is much appreciated. Several other "embarrassment" experts—in particular, Bill Cupach, Robert Edelmann, Andy Modigliani, and Jerry Parrott—were especially generous with information about (or reprint permissions for) their own work, and I am indebted to them as well.

The editorial and production staff at The Guilford Press were very gracious, and I value their kind help. Sam Houston State University has provided valued support for my studies of embarrassment for several years. Finally, the book profited from the keen inspection of Don Miller and Charlotte Miller; their contribution was very welcome.

ROWLAND S. MILLER
*Bryan, TX*

# Contents

# CHAPTER 1

# *The Nature*
# *of Embarrassment*

If you can read this book, you've been embarrassed. Your ability to comprehend these words depends on human qualities that far surpass those of most other species. You are intelligent and sophisticated enough to have a sense of personal identity that distinguishes you from other people. You possess capacities for introspection and self-knowledge that are marvelously complex. This humanity comes at a price, however: It makes you susceptible to embarrassment, an uncomfortable, aroused state of mortification, abashment, and chagrin that you can experience and lower animals cannot.

This book is a study of that uniquely human emotion. Embarrassment is, on the one hand, an ordinary, familiar emotion. The events that elicit it are sometimes dramatic and exotic—and we'll examine some accounts of embarrassment that are hilarious and others that are unsettling—but most embarrassments follow mundane, commonplace mishaps. The emotion itself is an experience most of us have encountered hundreds of times.

On the other hand, despite its familiarity, embarrassment is an emotion that holds rich, important insights into the social nature of humankind. Embarrassment depends on the existence of public self-consciousness, the ability to think about and be concerned with what other people are thinking about us, and this is an ability that few, if any, other species possess. It takes time for this special ability to develop; thus, unlike many other emotions, embarrassment does not exist at birth. As we will see, children may not experience the mature form of embarrassment familiar to adults until they gain both the socialization and the cognitive abilities of young adolescence.

Embarrassment is also an important component of social interaction throughout our lives. Early on, it's a valuable mechanism with which children can be taught the difference between right and wrong. Later, it's an indispensable tool that helps us redress our social sins. It enforces the standards that regulate our contact with our fellows, and embodies the pain and uncertainty we can feel when our expectations are violated. It's a familiar emotion *because* it plays such an important part in our interactions. It is far more important than you may realize.

Indeed, one way to gain a fuller appreciation of the functions and value of embarrassment is to imagine a person who cannot be embarrassed. Envision a fellow who, upon meeting a colleague's spouse for the first time at a cafeteria, spills a large soft drink from his tray onto her head.[1] She is seated at her table, and our protagonist is standing beside her. One moment a friendly introduction is being made—"Hello, it's a pleasure to meet . . ."—and the next, she has cola running down her back, dripping from her nose, and pooling in her lap. Now imagine that in response, our clumsy actor stays completely cool and calm, expressing regret but doing so with absolute aplomb. He is apologetic, but unemotional. Poised and unruffled, he offers to make financial amends, and then departs.

Later, you learn that this fellow has never been mortified or sheepish about anything he's ever done. He's immune to the practical jokes and teasing of his coworkers. He's untouched and unconcerned by anyone's evaluation of him. He simply doesn't care what people think. Do you like him? Can you trust him?

Contrast his preternatural poise with a more typical reaction to a drink spilled on the head of a new acquaintance. Imagine instead that our hero registers shock and chagrin and stammers out an abashed apology and offers of reparation while exhibiting obvious embarrassment.[2] Given that harm is done, who seems more likable, trustworthy, and kind, a person who does become embarrassed or one who does not?

When Gün Semin and Tony Manstead (1982) asked observers to make judgments much like these, they gave *poorer* ratings to a person who stayed too calm in an embarrassing situation; a person who was appropriately abashed was liked better. In fact, one remarkable fact about embarrassment that we will later examine in detail is that it is often a *desirable, correct* response to social predicaments. It is often an appropriate, useful response that helps make the best out of a bad situation.

We can even argue that it is abnormal to be immune to embarrassment, so that there's something unusual (or wrong) with someone who cannot be embarrassed. It's unbecoming and unseemly to dump a drink on someone's head with no apparent emotion. As W. R. Crozier (1990) colorfully suggested, "we might think that a person who is never embarrassed . . . is lacking some important human quality, is insensitive, thoughtless, or uncaring, a 'brazen hussy' or an 'arrogant son of a bitch' " (p. 7). A capacity for embarrassment is a marker of normal humanity, which makes it an intriguing emotion, indeed.

## CHARACTERISTICS OF EMBARRASSMENT

Let's characterize embarrassment further by considering another example. On a cool, drizzly day in central Texas, Marie, a 41-year-old graduate student at Texas A&M University, waited to cross a wide, busy street. She was running a bit late, and in her haste to get dressed she had donned an old maternity slip that was now too big for her. When the traffic finally came to a stop and she started across, the top of the slip slid down to her thighs. After a few more steps, it was around her knees, and, moments later, around her ankles. Rather than stop in front of five lanes of traffic to adjust the slip, or even gather it up, she decided, in the heat of embarrassment, to just step out of the slip and keep going. She shook her feet free, pulled her umbrella down around her face, picked up her pace, and left the slip lying in the street, a wasted garment and a sodden symbol of embarrassment.

This event may have been delightful for the drivers who witnessed it, and the hapless victim was able to laugh about it later on. Still, it was an unpleasant experience at the time, and, as a typical example of embarrassment, it can be instructive.

First, let's ponder her predicament. Clothes do fail us sometimes, and had her slip fallen to her shins while she was alone, she might have been annoyed, but not embarrassed. The fact that her predicament was public caused her a whole new set of concerns that would not have existed in private and that made embarrassment a possibility. People rarely seem to experience embarrassment when they are alone. It is a *social* emotion that depends on the real or imagined presence of others, and if people do experience "private" embarrassment when no else is present, it may be because they are vividly imagining what others would think had they been there.

Further, it is not important that we know those who observe us. As our heroine hurried across the street, she recognized no one and was unaware of anyone she particularly wanted to impress. The presence of mere strangers is enough to cause the discomfort of embarrassment, and we need not be sure that anyone is actually watching. Marie was embarrassed to find herself with her slip around her ankles even before anyone else could appear to notice. Moreover, her feelings did not result from any criticism from others that suggested that she looked foolish; later, she could not recall any reaction from those who may have witnessed her small mishap. Instead, her embarrassment depended on her knowledge that others, even total strangers, could notice her little misadventure, not that they already had. By the time we are adults, we do not need to be actually reproved by others to feel chagrin for our untoward or undesirable behavior. It is enough that we act in a manner that could allow others to form impressions of us that we would prefer them not to have, whether or not they seem to notice.

Now, consider Marie's response to her fallen slip. By leaving it behind, she was able to more quickly escape an awkward scene. She also avoided the further unwanted attention that might result from stopping and stooping to retrieve the lingerie. On the other hand, she abandoned a valuable garment, she littered the street, and she probably seemed doubly ridiculous to anyone who was really watching. How much more sensible it would have been simply to pause, collect the slip, shrug off the trivial judgments of strangers, and donate the slip to charity later on! Yet, a mature, competent woman did nothing of the sort. In the heat of the moment, it was more important to our heroine to escape her social predicament than it was to keep the slip. A remarkable aspect of embarrassment is that people often strive to avoid it, or to escape it once it has occurred, even when it is costly for them to do so.

In one demonstration of this point, Bert Brown (1970) asked college freshmen to perform, in private, either an awkward or an innocuous task. As part of a "sensory impressions" exercise, some of the students were asked to spend 3 minutes sucking, biting, and licking a baby's pacifier. Others merely handled and touched a small rubber soldier. Thereafter, the plot thickened; all the participants were asked to describe what they had done to an audience of fellow students in another room. Going public with these disclosures was likely to cause mild embarrassment to those students who had been sucking a pacifier, but several options were possible: The students could choose to write out an anonymous account of their sensations, create an audiotape that the audience would hear, make a videotape of their report, or actually meet the audience face to face. Brown's clever wrinkle was that the more publicity students accepted, the more money they would be paid for participating. Those who allowed personal public exposure of their actions received $1.50, whereas those who wished to maintain their privacy with a written report received no money at all.

The results of Brown's study demonstrated that people strive to avoid embarrassment even when they must make sacrifices to do so. The students who had "sensed" the pacifier, and who had more embarrassing actions to hide, chose to retain more privacy and accept less pay than did those who had handled the figure. In this investigation, people generally sought to avoid embarrassment even when it meant forgoing cold, hard cash. Indeed, in other real-life situations, the threat of embarrassment may be so aversive that people take risks or stomach real harm to avoid becoming embarrassed. For instance, Leary and Dobbins (1983) showed that adolescents who were embarrassed by the thought of buying contraceptives from a pharmacy were much less likely to use any contraception—but were no less sexually active—than their less embarrassable peers. Similarly, most people now know that condom usage can reduce their chances of catching the human immunodeficiency (or AIDS) virus, but lingering embarrassment associated with condoms is a stumbling block that keeps many from making the simple, smart choice to use one (Helwig-Larsen & Collins, 1994).

Thus, because they are so eager to avoid or escape it, people sometimes respond to embarrassment in disadvantageous ways. (With hindsight, Marie now wishes she had picked up her slip.) Embarrassment may also engender characteristic styles of behavior that reveal one's embarrassment to others. When she finally stepped out of her slip in the rainy intersection, Marie hid her face and scurried away, and even from a distance, observers may have been able to tell that she was less poised and relaxed. In fact, embarrassed people often engage in agitated, unique nonverbal behavior that shows others that they *are* embarrassed. Often, their body motion increases, they avert their gaze, smile sheepishly, and blush (Edelmann & Hampson, 1981a; Keltner, 1995). Importantly, such reactions mean that embarrassment is not only a social emotion that occurs in public, it is an *obvious* emotion that may be readily apparent to any others present.

Embarrassment's public nature has meaningful consequences. First of all, others may be able to reliably discern whether or not someone is embarrassed. Audiences may thus be reasonably certain whether a person is really chagrined by some misdeed, or implacable and unrepentant instead. Further, audiences may be able to detect embarrassment (especially as an obvious blush) even when someone wishes to conceal it. Second, because it is recognized by others, embarrassment may have a substantial effect on the interactions in which it occurs. Embarrassment is hardly ever ignored; it usually changes in some way the situation in which it occurs (Miller, 1995a). Bystanders may find themselves drawn into an embarrassed person's attempt to deal with his or her predicament. Realizing that someone is embarrassed, audiences may respond with compassionate support or hostile rejection, but only rarely do they fail to respond at all (Cupach & Metts, 1992). Someone else's discombobulation can easily become *our* awkward situation as everyone present struggles to get an interaction back on track. Were embarrassment simply an internal, private event, it would be more easily overlooked or ignored by others, and would be a less influential emotion.

Finally, as she scurried across the intersection, our heroine experienced the characteristic feelings of embarrassment. She felt conspicuous, foolish, awkward and uncomfortable, mortified and chagrined, all at once. Occurring as they did in the silly, public situation she faced, these feelings were unmistakable indications of embarrassment, and she had no doubt what emotion she was feeling at the time.

Still, when she was embarrassed, Marie was actually experiencing several different interrelated feelings, some of which also occur in other emotions. In feeling like a conspicuous center of attention, Marie was acutely aware that others were watching and judging her; she was in a state of "public self-awareness" and, at least for a moment, was especially concerned with what other people were thinking about her. This public self-awareness is one aspect of embarrassment that makes it a social emotion, but such self-awareness also underlies reactions such as shyness (the inhibition and anxiety that accompanies the prospect of interaction with others) and stage fright (anxiety associated with evaluation by an audience). In addition, her chagrin meant that Marie was distressed by this event; she regretted her behavior and was pained by it. Such unhappy contrition is also characteristic of shame and guilt.

Considering embarrassment in this light—as a mixture of several discrete sensations, some of which are not unique to embarrassment itself—has important implications for our understanding of its nature. One issue is conceptual. Recent debates among emotion researchers have contrasted two different means of categorizing emotions. On the one hand, we can define an emotional state with regard to a small set of essential features that characterize the emotion and that must be present for that emotion to occur. This classic approach assumes that emotions are discrete experiences that can be reliably and meaningfully discriminated from one another, and was the basis for early theories of emotion (such as Tomkins, 1962, 1963, and Izard, 1971; see Izard, 1993; Roseman, Wiest, & Swartz, 1994; and Scherer & Wallbott, 1994, for updates on discrete emotion theory). The classic approach argues for precision, and strives to pinpoint the necessary components of an experience that delineate it and unequivocally distinguish it from other emotions. This approach thus suggests that all experiences of embarrassment share certain key characteristics (or else embarrassment is not being felt, and some other emotion is occurring).

On the other hand, an alternative "prototype" approach argues that emotions are better understood not as clear-cut, disparate categories but as close, friendly neighbors who discourage fences between their yards

(Metts & Bowers, 1994). This view holds that people understand their emotional reactions by comparing them to idealized exemplars, or prototypes, of given emotions. These prototypes contain the features that exemplify a particular emotion, but acknowledge that certain features may or may not be present each time the emotion occurs. The identification of an experience as one emotion or another is thought to depend more on how closely a person's sensations *resemble*, rather than perfectly match, the set of characteristics that epitomize (but do not exclusively define) an emotion. In practice, this means that the boundaries between similar emotions may be rather imprecise. In addition, emotional experiences are not pure states that feel exactly the same every time. This view of emotions is not universally accepted (see Clore & Ortony, 1991), but it is now common for researchers to think of emotions as families of experiences that have fuzzy boundaries, rather than plain distinctions, between related emotional states (e.g., Russell, 1991; Russell & Fehr, 1994).

There are two consequences for our understanding of embarrassment in all this. First, the feelings that epitomize embarrassment may not necessarily be unique to embarrassment. Experiences that we casually apprehend as different emotions may have several features in common, and may sometimes be more similar to each other than they are different. In addition, any particular experience of embarrassment may not contain all the feelings that usually identify the emotion. Second, pinning down the precise differences between related emotions can be a tricky business. To the extent we understand our own diverse emotional experiences by comparing them to idealized prototypes, the perceived dividing line between related emotions may shift and change depending on the audience and situation we face and on the diligence with which we monitor our private, internal sensations.

We will expand on this second point in Chapter 2, when we distinguish embarrassment from its closest neighbor, shame. For now, let's note that even if we do use prototypes to identify our emotions, our emotion knowledge is not *that* inexact. Most of us possess a reasonably well-articulated concept of embarrassment that allows us to recognize clearly whether or not we're embarrassed. Moreover, a common prototype of embarrassment may be widely shared by members of a given culture.

## PROTOTYPICAL EMBARRASSMENT

Jerry Parrott and Stefanie Smith (1991) assessed our shared understanding of embarrassment by asking 121 Georgetown University students to write detailed accounts of either a real incident they had found embarrassing or, instead, what generally happens to most people when they become embarrassed. Parrott and Smith thus obtained the students' beliefs about *typical* episodes of embarrassment and were able to compare them to dozens of reports of *actual* embarrassment that others had really experienced.

In general, there was substantial agreement between the two types of accounts. Embarrassment was believed to result from various events in which people lost control of a situation and appeared inconsistent, inappropriate, or incongruous to the other people present. As a result of such events, people felt foolish, inept, awkward, and uncomfortable; they felt exposed, like the center of attention, and worried about what others were thinking. They often blushed. In response to these incidents, they tried either to explain themselves, make a joke of the incident, ignore it nervously, or to escape the predicament by leaving. Other people sometimes became involved in these repair efforts, aiding and abetting a person's attempt to laugh it off or ignore it.

These characteristics fit the examples of embarrassment we have encountered thus far, and appear to be reliable exemplars of embarrassment. Interestingly, however, Parrott and Smith (1991) found that their subjects' beliefs about embarrassment did not always coincide with the actual episodes they described. Although people's conceptions of typical embarrassment fit memories of actual embarrassment reasonably well, there were several reliable differences between the global conceptions and the real events. In particular, subjects conceived of typical embarrassment as resulting from real failure or wrongdoing on the part of the embarrassed person, whereas those remembering actual embarrassments were more likely to think of themselves as the victims of adverse events. As Parrott and Smith noted, remembered accounts of real personal embarrassment seemed to stem "less from personal failure than from helplessness, entrapment, or a lack of social manoeuvrability" (p. 484). Remembered embarrassments were more surprising and unavoidable and less controllable than hypothetical, "typical" embarrassments were.

Other, more specific differences between the "typical" and "actual" accounts were also interesting. All of the remembered episodes of real embarrassment occurred when other people were present, but a few people believed that embarrassment could occur without any audience at all. Blushing was widely believed to be characteristic of embarrassment, but was mentioned by only three-fifths of those describing real predicaments. Once embarrassment occurred, people tried to cope in a variety of different ways, so that no one particular response was as typical as people tended to think it was.

These various discrepancies are noted in Table 1.1, which lists the frequency with which Parrott and Smith's (1991) respondents reported

**TABLE 1.1. Features of Prototypical Embarrassment**

| Specific features | Frequency of mention in accounts of | |
| --- | --- | --- |
| | "Typical" embarrassment | Actual embarrassment |
| **The predicaments** | | |
| Other people present* | 93% | 100% |
| Making bad impression* | 64% | 44% |
| Contradicting desired identity or image* | 54% | 79% |
| Seeming incongruous or out of place* | 43% | 19% |
| Private or intimate matters revealed | 36% | 26% |
| Situation out of control* | 31% | 56% |
| Subject to ridicule or laughter* | 23% | 40% |
| **The feelings** | | |
| Blushing* | 89% | 58% |
| Awkward, uncomfortable, nervous | 49% | 53% |
| Desire to hide or escape* | 44% | 25% |
| Foolish, inferior, incompetent | 41% | 47% |
| Concerned about others' judgments | 39% | 32% |
| Center of attention* | 31% | 56% |
| **The responses** | | |
| Leaving or escaping* | 48% | 28% |
| Changing subject* | 44% | 0% |
| Saying nothing | 36% | 28% |
| Making a joke of it* | 33% | 16% |
| Providing excuses* | 33% | 12% |
| Looking away, hiding face | 31% | 18% |

*Note.* The data are drawn from "Embarrassment: Actual vs. Typical Cases, Classical vs. Prototypical Representations," by W. G. Parrott and S. F. Smith, 1991, *Cognition and Emotion, 5*, pp. 479–480. Copyright 1991 by Lawrence Erlbaum Associates Limited. Reprinted by permission of Erlbaum (UK) Taylor & Francis, Hove, UK. Items with an asterisk denote meaningful distinctions between the memories of actual embarrassment and the imagined episodes of "typical" embarrassment.

particular characteristics of both "typical" and real embarrassment. I think that two aspects of the results in the table are of interest. First, the occasional disparities between envisioned "typical" embarrassment and memories of the real thing demonstrate that, just as suspected, our prototypes aren't perfect. The representations of customary embarrassment that come to mind as standards of comparison have good, but not perfect, fit with the actual episodes of embarrassment we are likely to recall. Thus, as I have suggested, scientific caution about the precision of the concepts with which people identify and distinguish their emotions is warranted.

Second, however, despite the limits imposed by "fuzzy boundaries" and individual idiosyncrasy, we do share widespread agreement about the nature of embarrassment. Table 1.1 shows that people's personal prototypes of embarrassment are remarkably similar, sharing particular features and symptoms to a striking degree. The conspicuous consensus about "typical" embarrassment is especially impressive because Parrott and Smith (1991) obtained open-ended accounts of embarrassment that did not suggest exactly what the respondents should say; therefore, the frequencies listed in Table 1.1 describe the proportion of respondents who thought of a particular feature, and considered it to be characteristic of embarrassment, on their own. In that light, any symptom or feature that came to mind for even a third of the respondents is notable, because memories aren't perfect and it's very easy for people to overlook specific points of general events they are asked to recall (Linton, 1982).

The bottom line is that hundreds of people have now been asked to detail their experiences of embarrassment in this (Parrott & Smith, 1991) and other studies (e.g., Miller, 1992; Tangney, Miller, Flicker, & Barlow, 1996), and central themes always emerge. Embarrassment *is* that state of awkward abashment and chagrin that results from public events that disrupt our expectations and communicate unwanted impressions of ourselves to others. It is an uncomfortable emotion that will be avoided if possible. Moreover, if it does occur, embarrassment engenders characteristic physical and behavioral reactions, and usually motivates attempts to repair or escape the awkward situation. We do know what embarrassment feels like, we don't like it, and we avoid it when we can.

## A LOOK AHEAD

Embarrassment may be a familiar, recognizable emotion, but there is still much to understand. In coming chapters, I will examine the origins and effects of embarrassment in detail. I'll trace the development and emergence of embarrassment in childhood, and inspect personality differences in susceptibility to embarrassment. I will establish a comprehensive catalogue of embarrassing predicaments, and explain why such events cause us pain. I'll also explore the consequences and outcomes of embarrassment in interaction, and consider strategies for coping with embarrassment.

We'll find that this intriguing emotion is important for several reasons. First, it is normal to be embarrassable, and embarrassment is widespread, occurring around the world in Eastern, as well as Western, cultures (Sueda & Wiseman, 1992). It's a prevalent emotion; most young adults are embarrassed by something each and every week (Stonehouse & Miller, 1994). More importantly, embarrassment is influential. The desire to avoid embarrassment and to reduce it once it occurs pervades our social behavior, and embarrassment serves meaningful functions in social life.

Before we can address such issues, however, we need to clear one more definitional hurdle. We may share a coherent prototype of embarrassment and generally understand its nature, but still encounter difficulty in precisely distinguishing it from a close neighbor, such as shame. In fact, the distinctions among embarrassment, shame, and other related emotions have been poorly realized by most scholars. For that reason, and because our goal is to understand embarrassment as fully as possible, I'll explicate those distinctions in the next chapter.

CHAPTER 2

# Embarrassment
# as a Basic Emotion

We have established that people generally share similar conceptions of
embarrassment, widely agreeing on the experiences that characterize the
emotion (Parrott & Smith, 1991). However, we have also found that
there are few features of embarrassment that are universally acknowledged to typify the state; no one characteristic of embarrassment was
always mentioned by people who were asked to "describe what generally
happens when people feel embarrassed" (Parrott & Smith, 1991, pp.
470–471). Such imprecision does not necessarily imply that our ability
to identify embarrassment is faulty. After all, the features of embarrassment listed in Table 1.1 were generated from memory, and people who
are actually experiencing embarrassment may be much more precise.
Nonetheless, if people do use prototypes to identify their emotions, there
may be some variability in individuals' comprehension of their experiences. In addition, the boundaries between closely related emotions may
be indistinct, so that there are few obvious differences between similar
emotions for either introspection or careful observation to specify.

For these reasons, a good test of our practical knowledge of embarrassment lies in the facility with which we are able to differentiate
embarrassment from other emotional states. As we experience them
ourselves, the differences between related emotions may be relative
rather than abrupt. Therefore, if it is attainable, the ability to reliably
differentiate embarrassment from its neighbors would suggest that people understand embarrassment reasonably well.

The best example of all this with regard to embarrassment involves the distinctions between embarrassment and what is probably its closest neighbor, shame. Until recently, a common assumption was either that there were *no* important distinctions between the two emotions, or that, if they were different, embarrassment was simply a milder, less intense version of shame. Of course, if that were so, there would be no persuasive reason to write a whole book on embarrassment; one could simply write a book on shame and note that everything said therein applies to embarrassment, but to a milder degree. As you can guess, because I *am* writing a book just on embarrassment, I don't think embarrassment is synonymous with shame at all. To the contrary, recent research argues that embarrassment *is* a singular, unique emotion that can be distinguished in fundamental ways from related states. Indeed, it may even be one of a small group of primary, "basic" emotions that address rudimentary human needs. These issues warrant some discussion, however, so this chapter addresses the differences among embarrassment, shame, and other related emotions.

## BASIC EMOTIONS

One widely shared perspective on emotion presumes that there are a few emotions that are distinctive enough, both in phenomenology and physical effects, to be understood as one of perhaps 10 or 11 "basic" emotions that occur in human beings. Paul Ekman (1992) has persuasively argued that a few discrete emotions are indispensable, key human reactions because they, first, occur in all of us, across all cultures, and, second, have had adaptive, valuable benefits in helping us deal with "fundamental life-tasks." These tasks are the "universal human predicaments, such as achievements, losses, frustrations, etc." (Ekman, p. 171) that all of us face, and the basic emotions gradually evolved among our ancestors, according to Ekman, because they helped people cope effectively with these common dilemmas. Basic emotions fulfilled the useful function of mobilizing quick, adaptive reactions to "important interpersonal encounters" (Ekman, p. 171), and those with a ready repertoire of appropriate emotions were presumably more likely to survive the harsh environments of our tribal past than were those who were emotionally inept. Natural selection may thus have promoted the spread of certain especially useful fundamental emotions.

"Basic" emotions, then, would be a core group of discrete emotions of special importance and consequence. The belief that there are such emotions has been the central theme of the work of several influential theorists. Sylvan Tomkins (1962, 1963) believed that there were 9 basic emotions that were innate, being encoded into specific areas of the brain. Carroll Izard (1971, 1977) enumerated 10 fundamental emotions: fear, anger, joy, disgust, interest, surprise, contempt, shame, sadness, and guilt. Robert Plutchik (1980) counted only 8 basic emotions, but described how many different, "mixed" emotions could result from combinations of the 8. The most specific criteria for distinguishing the basic emotions from complex, blended, or mixed emotions such as jealousy or scorn, however, were offered by Ekman (1992), who argued that fundamental emotions possess several particular characteristics.

First, Ekman argued that such emotions evidence (1) quick onset, (2) brief duration, and (3) unbidden occurrence. They occur involuntarily, and we do not choose when to experience them. They arise very quickly but last for only minutes or seconds, not hours or days. In addition, such emotions are thought to depend on some process of (4) relatively automatic appraisal in which a triggering stimulus is recognized almost instantly, without a lot of conscious analysis. As a result, compelling events can elicit basic emotional responses before we have given them any thought or decided what to do.

These first four criteria distinguish emotions from other feeling states (such as moods, which are less specific and do last for extended periods of time) and are thought to typify all emotions. However, Ekman believed three further characteristics are found only in basic emotions. One of these is (5) universal antecedent events. Because they presumably evolved to help us manage shared fundamental problems, basic emotions spring from recognizably similar situations around the world. Cultural variation is to be expected, but the same general events that elicit a basic emotion in one group of people should rouse similar responses elsewhere, as well. Basic emotions should also be accompanied by (6) distinctive physiological responses, exhibiting unique patterns of autonomic nervous system activity and other such physical markers. Finally, for Ekman, "the strongest evidence for distinguishing one emotion from another" (1992, p. 175) comes from (7) distinctive universal signals of an emotion in the form of facial expression and behavior. Basic emotions are reflected in a singular facial display that constitutes an emblematic, recognizable signal to other people that the emotion is taking place.

Ekman also offered the possibility that some basic emotions were (8) present in other animals, but was more tentative about this characteristic because some emotions might have emerged only in humans. He also acknowledged leaving the subjective experience of an emotion— "how each emotion feels" (1992, p. 175)—off his list, saying that more information was needed about the links between subjective experience and the other components of emotional response. However, characteristic thoughts and feelings, such as the sensations of foolish awkwardness that accompany embarrassment, do reliably distinguish emotions from one another (Lazarus, 1991; Roseman et al., 1994), and should probably be added to the list.

## EMBARRASSMENT'S STATUS

When they were constructing their lists of basic emotions, none of the theorists mentioned above included embarrassment in that group. Ekman (1992) came closest, admitting that "when the research is completed" (p. 191) he expected embarrassment to have all the characteristics he described. Of course, much more *is* known now, and I think that embarrassment is unquestionably a basic emotion.[1]

It is certainly typified by the rapid, involuntary, and relatively automatic onset that characterizes all emotions. When I accidentally dumped a large soft drink onto the head of a new acquaintance (see Chapter 1), I was seized by embarrassment before I had a chance to ponder my situation. I was embarrassed before I knew it, and my emotion did not depend on a thoughtful analysis of the predicament I was in. In addition, although I was profoundly embarrassed, that first intense flash of mortification and chagrin waned considerably within a few minutes. The memory was humiliating (and it still makes me cringe), but the overwhelming tidal wave of feeling faded fast. Embarrassment thus possesses all of the general characteristics of emotion, and everyone agrees that embarrassment is an emotional response (e.g., Shaver, Schwartz, Kirson, & O'Connor, 1987).

But is it a *basic* emotion? Recent evidence suggests that it is. The variety of events that cause embarrassment (which we catalogue in Chapter 4) elicit similar distressed reactions in different cultures around the world (as is documented in Chapter 6). Embarrassment does seem to have universal antecedent events. In addition, it is usually accompanied by a unique pattern of nonverbal behavior that distinguishes it from other emotions, and that makes a person's embarrassment obvious to others. Embarrassed people shrink from others by looking away, turning their heads, touching their faces, and controlling their smiles; we'll describe these distinctive universal signals of embarrassment in Chapter 8.

Less is known about the precise physical responses that may distinguish embarrassment from other emotions, but that is mostly due to the complex nature of research in this area (Cacioppo, Klein, Berntson, & Hatfield, 1993; Levenson, 1992). Differences may lurk in blood pressure, heart rate, skin conductance, muscular tension, respiration, finger temperature, pulse transit time, and a variety of other measures. In addition, emotional responses may be mediated either by the sympathetic nervous system, which energizes the body for action by increasing heart rate, respiration, and perspiration, or by the parasympathetic nervous system, which slows activity by reducing heart rate and blood pressure and stimulating digestion. Embarrassment may be unusually complex, involving both branches of the nervous system in an intricate response.

On the one hand, people feel tense and aroused when they get embarrassed (Miller & Fahey, 1991), and their fingers get cooler as blood is diverted away from the skin (Leary, Rejeski, Britt, & Smith, 1994); these are effects of sympathetic activation. On the other hand, embarrassed people often blush as the flow of blood to the face increases (Drummond, 1989), and their heart rates normally decrease (Buck & Parke, 1972); these are parasympathetic responses. Leary and his colleagues speculated that embarrassment routinely involves both sympathetic and parasympathetic effects, as people are aroused by their predicaments but often frozen into immobility as they try to shrink and hide from their humiliating plights. When embarrassment strikes, we may behave like deer paralyzed by oncoming headlights; we can be very upset at the same time that we feel stupefied and uncertain, unable to respond resourcefully to a surprising threat.

Leary, Rejeski, et al. (1994) obtained this pattern when they embarrassed young women at Wake Forest University by measuring the body fat around their thighs and waists. Some of the women were surprised by this procedure; almost before they knew it, an experimenter was placing calipers around a pinch of skin on the side of their waists. Other women were forewarned about the procedure and had time to sit and think about it before it began. Various physiological measures were obtained throughout the study, and those who had time to ponder the upcoming assessment were obviously aroused by their predicament. As they prepared to face the embarrassing event, their heart rates and diastolic blood pressures increased, a response typical of anxious, "fight-or-flight," sympathetic activation. Once the measurements began, however, their heart rates and diastolic pressures decreased, and their facial temperatures increased, reflecting parasympathetic control. Once the calipers were applied, the women could do little but sit there mortified, and they seemed to "freeze and hide" physically. Responses to a foreseen embarrassment thus came in two phases; the first was predominantly sympathetic arousal (much like anxiety) but the second was chiefly parasympathetic withdrawal (which does not occur in anxiety states at all).

In contrast, those who were surprised by the physical exam—whose embarrassment was unexpected, like most of the embarrassments we encounter in daily life—exhibited this sympathetic surprise and parasympathetic withdrawal in quicker succession. Their responses were more mixed and more complex. Leary and his colleagues suggested that, at bottom, the physiological reactions a person displays in response to an embarrassing predicament may depend on the level of threat he or she perceives. If the predicament seems escapable or reparable, sympathetic responses may remain foremost as the person actively copes with the situation. On the other hand, if the difficulty is inescapable and must be helplessly endured, the sinking feelings of parasympathetic retreat may dominate.

In any case, the general pattern of embarrassment's physiological underpinnings—cooler hands, warmer faces, variable heart rate, increases in skin conductance (Leary, Rejeski, et al., 1994; Miller & Fahey, 1991)—is relatively unusual (A. H. Buss, 1980), and at least one response is quite unique: blushing. We will consider blushing in some detail in Chapter 8, but, for now, we can note that all by itself it may meet Ekman's (1992) criteria of both a distinctive physiological response and a distinctive universal signal.

Embarrassment may also have a relatively unique home in the brain. Many other emotions are regulated by the limbic system, a collection of structures just above the brainstem that control other processes, such as hunger and thirst, that we share with other animals (LeDoux, 1995). However (as Chapter 5 will demonstrate), embarrassment depends on the complex capacity for self-consciousness that is found only in other primates and that emerges from the more advanced regions of the brain known as the cerebral cortex (the wrinkled outer layer of the brain). Unlike many other emotions, embarrassment depends on the same areas of the brain in which our conscious thought occurs, the prefrontal cortex (Cutlip & Leary, 1993). People lose the capacity for embarrassment when the medial frontal lobe of the cortex is damaged (Devinsky, Hafler, & Victor, 1982), and damage in that region would be unlikely to change a person's capacity for other emotions such as anger or fear.

Overall, then, our emerging understanding of embarrassment's physiology supports the possibility that embarrassment has a unique physical signature. Some data are tentative, but it appears that the only one of Ekman's (1992) criteria for basic emotions that embarrassment does not meet is "presence in other animals." Because it requires the rare, complicated, self-conscious ability to envision what others are thinking of us (as Chapter 7 will assert), embarrassment occurs only in humans and, conceivably, the great apes (see Gallup, 1977, 1979). Regardless of what pet owners may believe, embarrassment does not exist in dogs, cats, rabbits, parrots, or iguanas. (Dog owners who think their animals look embarrassed are probably mistaking fear or confusion for self-conscious chagrin.) In fact, there is no firm evidence that suggests that embarrassment occurs in any other species than our own. If this is true, it violates Ekman's expectation that basic emotions should be shared by diverse species because they address fundamental survival needs. On the other hand, because of humanity's special qualities, it's not unreasonable to expect some basic emotions in people that do *not* occur in other animals. As Lazarus (1991) argued, some emotions such as embarrassment, shame, guilt, and regret "may have emerged on the basis of greater human cognitive and social complexity, and . . . may be unique to humans . . . but no less primary in the process of survival" (p. 81).

Thus, on the whole, recent studies of embarrassment indicate that it probably is a basic emotion. At this point, few scholars recognize it as such, however, for two reasons; first, they haven't studied embarrassment in much detail, and second, they're not sure that embarrassment is reliably different from shame, another emotion that some theorists (Izard, 1977; Tomkins, 1963) *do* believe to be basic. To fully appreciate embarrassment's uniqueness, we need to distinguish it from other social concerns such as shyness and stage fright in general, and from shame in particular.

## EMBARRASSMENT'S NEIGHBORS

There are several types of anxiety and nervousness that people experience in social situations; collectively, they are all instances of *social anxiety*, or apprehension, trepidation, or fear that arise from "the prospect or presence of interpersonal evaluation in real or imagined social settings" (Leary & Kowalski, 1995, p. 6). The specific situations that create such qualms are diverse, and researchers often distinguish among dating anxiety, public speaking anxiety (or stage fright), and shyness, as well as others. However, the primary emotion in all of these states is anxiety. They are not discrete emotions; they differ only in the social context in which they occur, and not in the subjective sensations people encounter.

Accordingly, researchers have found it useful to classify the conditions that cause concern about others' evaluations. Two distinctions can be made (P. R. Harris, 1990; Leary & Kowalski, 1995; Schlenker & Leary, 1982). First, dread of others' judgments is often "anticipatory," occurring before anything actually goes wrong, whereas, on other occasions, it is "reactive," arising after unwanted events have already occurred. Second, the interpersonal encounters that trigger evaluative concern are sometimes "contingent" interactions in which our behavior depends on the responses of others, or, on other occasions, "noncontingent" performances in which our actions are largely predetermined.

The first distinction is particularly important in distinguishing embarrassment from these other states (P. R. Harris, 1990; Leary &

Kowalski, 1995). From this perspective, social anxiety is ordinarily anticipatory, with the sufferer worrying about undesired evaluations that have yet to occur. Thus, people can fret long in advance of an upcoming date or speech, and the events that cause social anxiety are rarely unexpected. In contrast, embarrassment is reactive, typically following unexpected events that have already, suddenly, created the real potential for unwanted judgments from others. Being anticipatory, social anxiety involves sympathetic nervous system arousal as people prepare for a threatening experience with increased heart rate and perspiration, and faster breathing (Leary & Kowalski, 1995). In contrast, as we have seen, embarrassed responses include a substantial parasympathetic component once a threatening event has already occurred (A. H. Buss, 1980; Leary, Rejeski, et al., 1994).

In addition, the "contingency" distinction can differentiate among several social anxieties, but it's not much help in understanding embarrassment. For instance, contingent interactions create dating anxiety and shyness, whereas noncontingent performances engender stage fright (Schlenker & Leary, 1982). However, both types of situations can readily cause embarrassment (as we will demonstrate in Chapter 4). Whether we are performing alone or engaged in conversation, unwanted events that threaten our "social identities," our images in the eyes of others, can precipitate embarrassment.

At bottom, however, the key distinction between the social anxieties and embarrassment is that they are simply different emotions. Regardless of the situations that trigger them, the social anxieties are all grounded in the same agitated apprehensiveness, fear, and dread: They are all instances of anxiety. Embarrassment is often considered to be related to the social anxieties (Leary & Kowalski, 1995) because it emerges from a similar social foundation of acute concerns about what others must be thinking. It is not a state of anxiety, however (P. R. Harris, 1990); it involves startled surprise and mortification, which are wholly absent in anxiety states per se.

Let's provide an illustration by comparing embarrassment to shyness, a prevalent social syndrome with which it is sometimes confused (Crozier, 1990). Properly speaking, shyness is not an emotion at all. Instead, it is a syndrome in which social anxiety is paired with awkward and inhibited social behavior (Cheek & Briggs, 1990; Leary & Kowalski, 1995). People who tend to be shy feel tense and worried during social interactions and display reticent, withdrawn, defensive behavior. Importantly, they also doubt themselves. Shy people believe they have a low level of social skill, and they lack confidence that they can manage their interactions satisfactorily (Cheek & Melchior, 1990; Miller, 1995b). Thus, shyness is defined by a particular pattern of anxiety *and* behavior that emerges from a characteristic habit of pessimistic thought and negative self-appraisal.

In contrast, embarrassment has little to do with what we think of ourselves, and it is not defined by any one type of interactive behavior. People's responses to an embarrassing predicament may be quite diverse, as we will see in Chapter 9. Further, a person's susceptibility to embarrassment is not much affected by that person's global levels of social skill or self-esteem (Miller, 1995b). Instead, if a sufficiently surprising and dramatic event confounds our expectations and arouses the threat of unwanted evaluations from others, almost any of us will respond with flustered abashment and chagrin, which is a discrete emotional response distinct from anxiety.

Individual proclivities toward shyness and embarrassment share common origins in awareness of and concern for what others think of us. Beyond that shared foundation, however, the two are quite different. Shyness involves anticipatory anxiety whereas embarrassment consists of reactive surprise and fluster. Shyness is a more fearful experience whereas embarrassment is more surprising, less enjoyable, more anger provoking, and more shameful (Mosher & White, 1981).

## DIFFERENTIATING EMBARRASSMENT AND SHAME

It may be harder to distinguish embarrassment from shame because they seem (to some people) to have so much in common. Indeed, diverse scholars have believed there to be no meaningful difference between the two emotions. Philosophers have asserted that embarrassment is merely "a euphemism for shame" (English, 1975, p. 25), and psychodynamic theorists have argued that "however mild or intense, embarrassment is not a different affect" (Kaufman, 1989, p. 24). More elaborate analyses by emotion specialists have usually allowed that shame is stronger than embarrassment, but have often suggested that the two are otherwise very similar (see Frijda, 1986). For instance, Richard Lazarus (1991) considered embarrassment an "alternative term" for shame (p. 244) but did note that, compared to shame, embarrassment seems "rather mild" (p. 245).

If embarrassment and shame really are just stronger and weaker forms of the same emotion, then distinguishing them would be tricky, indeed. The boundary between them could be arbitrary and shifting, and the difference between them hard to discern. However, a few other scholars have suggested possible reasons why shame is more intense than embarrassment, and, collectively, these suppositions propose differences between the emotions that are more meaningful.

## Proposed Differences

Arnold Buss (1980) argued that shame is more severe because it has "moral implications" (p. 162) that embarrassment does not have. According to Buss, a breach of a fundamental standard of conduct causes shame, whereas a minor breach of manners or poise causes embarrassment. Public revelation of relatively awful actions such as cowardly failing to render emergency aid to an accident victim, or infecting a spouse with a sexually transmitted disease caught from a prostitute, would presumably cause shame, not embarrassment. This idea has since been echoed by others. Ortony, Clore, and Collins asserted that "in order to feel shame, one must have violated a standard one takes to be *important*, as moral standards are" (1988, p. 142). Lewis (1992) concurred, arguing that "failures associated with less important, less central standards, rules, and goals result in embarrassment rather than shame" (p. 82). Harré eloquently suggested that "shame is appropriate in cases of serious derelictions that would, if publicly noticed, lead to assessments of character so unfavourable as to permanently depreciate one's honour. Embarrassment is the emotion proper to the violation of mere convention, a code of manners" (1990, p. 197). None of this should be taken to suggest that embarrassment is trivial. (Indeed, embarrassment may occur much more often, and thereby be a larger influence on daily life.) Nevertheless, these theorists all suggested that the two emotions occur in wholly different situations that should help us tell them apart.

Shame may also be more intense because of the interpersonal consequences that follow such transgressions. Behavior that produces shame may create more damning impressions in the eyes of others, implying that a person has defects in personality, morals, or character that are not evident when one becomes embarrassed (A. H. Buss, 1980; Shott, 1979). Whereas embarrassment may be more associated with accidents, mistakes, and goofs, shame may suggest the existence of lasting, intrinsic, personal faults. Shameful behavior would thus cause more, and more lasting, damage to a person's social identity. Both emotions may result from events that communicate unwanted images of oneself to others, but the impressions associated with shame may be more negative and less forgivable. As a part of this, the attributions of blame that others generate for the two emotions are likely to differ as well. Shame may typically follow misbehavior that is judged to be relatively internal, stable, and global in origin, whereas embarrassment is excused as more external, temporary, and limited in extent (G. Taylor, 1985).

The two emotions probably *feel* different, too, beyond one simply being stronger than the other. A. H. Buss (1980) asserted that, because their transgressions are more trivial and temporary, embarrassed people feel foolish whereas shameful people are regretful and depressed. In addition, shame probably contains more guilt and fear than embarrassment does (Mosher & White, 1981).

Finally, it is possible that shame has private effects that embarrassment does not have. In Chapter 7, I'll argue that embarrassment is fundamentally based on our concerns about what others are thinking of us; as a result, it depends on the presence of a real or imagined audience (Edelmann, 1994; Leary & Meadows, 1991) and doesn't have much to do with what we think of ourselves (Miller, 1995b, 1996). Shame may involve larger changes in self-evaluation and self-recrimination. Because it follows more meaningful immoralities, shame may cause momentary losses of self-esteem that do not occur in embarrassment (A. H. Buss, 1980). Moreover, because those drops in self-esteem may occur whether or not anyone else knows about our misbehavior, we may be able to feel shame even when others have no knowledge of our sins. Conceivably, then, unlike embarrassment, "shame can be an entirely internal experience with no one else present" (Kaufman, 1989, p. 6). Thus, shame may occur in both public and private conditions (a notion accepted by both Lewis, 1992, and Ortony et al., 1988).

However, this and the earlier suppositions about embarrassment and shame are merely speculative. Although there is general agreement that shame is a grimmer emotion that has more weighty effects, none of the foregoing theorists provided any empirical data to support their suppositions. Furthermore, disagreements existed. For example, some observers asserted that embarrassment could also occur in private when no one else was around, simply because an important personal standard was violated (Babcock, 1988).

### Some Research at Last

This was the intellectual situation June Tangney and I faced when we decided to attempt a detailed comparison of embarrassment and shame. We were dealing with two emotions arguably more alike than different, following in the footsteps of some scholars who saw meaningful distinctions between them and others who perceived few, if any, differences at all. There were only two prior studies to build on. Manstead and Tetlock (1989) had obtained global ratings of the situations that produce shame and embarrassment and found them to be quite similar; however, their respondents did report feeling less responsibility for embarrassment than for shame, and they considered embarrassment to be more unpredictable. Mosher and White (1981) had asked subjects to rate remembered shame and embarrassment experiences on Izard's (1977) Differential Emotions Scale, and found that embarrassment entailed more surprise and less fear, guilt, disgust, and anger than shame did. These findings were consistent with some of the hypothesized distinctions discussed above, but they obviously left several suppositions unexplored.

June Tangney, from George Mason University, is an expert on shame who had developed a personality measure to assess individual susceptibility to shame, and her work suggested that shame was a much uglier, darker emotion than embarrassment (Tangney, 1990, 1991, 1995). Shame makes people angry at both themselves and others; when they are feeling shame, people lack empathy for others and tend to be malicious and self-serving. Further, Tangney had found that people whose personalities make them prone to shame also tend to display various forms of psychological maladjustment. Shame-prone adults tend to be depressed and anxious (Tangney, Wagner, & Gramzow, 1992), and shame-prone children exhibit low self-esteem, poor self-control, and excessive hostility (Tangney, Burggraf, & Wagner, 1995). From what she had learned, we didn't think that embarrassment was much like shame at all.

To pinpoint the distinctions between the two emotions, we asked 104 college students to recall three situations that caused them embarrassment, and three other, different situations in which their strongest feeling was shame (Miller & Tangney, 1994). They were asked to reconstruct these experiences as vividly as possible and were encouraged to relive what they were thinking, feeling, and doing at the time. Then, with these recollections fresh in their minds, they were given cards that each contained a statement hypothesized to exemplify one of the emotions, and asked to sort each card into either a "Shame" or an "Embarrassment" stack. The statements embodied our own and others' assumptions about the emotions, and the participants were instructed to adjust their choices as often as necessary until they were content.

At no point did we define or describe either emotion for the participants; we were interested in the distinctions people used themselves. And, reflecting people's fuzzy prototypes and the neighborly similarity of the two emotions, none of the statements was unanimously understood to characterize one emotion better than the other. Nevertheless, most of the statements were judged to fit embarrassment better than shame, or vice versa, by large majorities of the participants. Despite the idiosyncrasies of the remembered experiences, clear patterns emerged, and the differences listed in Tables 2.1 and 2.2 are so large, there's less than 0.1% probability that they could have occurred by chance.

The statements are listed in the tables with regard to the size of the majorities that grouped them with each emotion. As you can see, the two emotions were remembered quite differently. Light-hearted, funny predicaments were almost always embarrassing rather than shameful. People often found embarrassments to be "kind of humorous" and said they smiled and "felt like laughing" at themselves. In contrast, people recalling shameful episodes "took the situation very seriously," felt angry with themselves, and did not smile. Whereas people often made jokes about embarrassing predicaments, they rarely laughed off shameful situations; instead, they apologized and "tried to make things better." The greater gravity of shameful situations was also reflected by others' responses to the event. Embarrassed people recalled that observers had been laughing at them, but shameful people thought that "other people were disgusted with me."

TABLE 2.1. Descriptors of Embarrassment

| Descriptor | Proportion of participants |
|---|---|
| The situation was kind of humorous. | 93% |
| I smiled. | 92% |
| I felt like laughing at myself. | 90% |
| I tried to make a joke about it. | 89% |
| I felt that other people were laughing at me. | 89% |
| There were other people around. | 89% |
| The feeling lasted a short time. | 86% |
| It only bothered me because other people were around or knew about it. | 83% |
| The situation was surprising to me. | 78% |
| The feeling hit me very quickly. | 77% |
| I tried to get out of the situation as soon as possible. | 76% |
| It was an accident. | 74% |
| I felt awkward. | 73% |
| The feeling was somewhat mild. | 72% |
| The feeling was caused by a temporary error. | 71% |
| I kept worrying about what others were thinking. | 70% |

*Note.* The percentages denote the number of participants who agreed that the statement described embarrassment better than shame. Each is statistically significant, indicating a better fit with embarrassment by at least $p < .001$. The data are from "Differentiating Embarrassment and Shame," by R. S. Miller and J. P. Tangney, 1994, *Journal of Social and Clinical Psychology, 13*, pp. 282–283. Copyright 1994 by The Guilford Press. Reprinted by permission.

Other people seemed to play different roles in shaping the two emotions as well. Embarrassed people tended to keep "worrying about what others were thinking," and were distressed only because "other people were around or knew about it." By comparison, people recalling shame often said they had been alone and that they had learned something they hadn't wanted to know about themselves. Whereas embarrassment seemed to depend on public exposure, shame often seemed to include a person's painful realization of his or her own imperfections. This suggests that shame does have a private component that does not exist in embarrassment, perhaps because self-evaluation (as opposed to social evaluation from others) plays a larger role in shame.

**TABLE 2.2. Descriptors of Shame**

| Descriptor | Proportion of participants |
| --- | --- |
| I felt like a bad person. | 91% |
| I did not smile. | 82% |
| I felt angry with myself. | 82% |
| I learned something I didn't want to know about myself. | 82% |
| The feeling developed over time. | 82% |
| I felt I was immoral. | 81% |
| I took the situation very seriously. | 80% |
| Afterwards, I apologized. | 79% |
| I felt that other people were disgusted with me. | 79% |
| The feeling lasted a long time. | 78% |
| It was no accident. | 73% |
| The feeling was caused by a deep-seated flaw. | 72% |
| I was alone. | 68% |
| I saw the situation coming in some way. | 65% |
| Afterwards, I tried to make things better. | 65% |
| The feeling was very strong. | 65% |

*Note.* The percentages denote the number of participants who agreed that the statement described shame better than embarrassment. Each is statistically significant, indicating a better fit with shame by at least $p < .001$. The data are from "Differentiating Embarrassment and Shame," by R. S. Miller and J. P. Tangney, 1994, *Journal of Social and Clinical Psychology, 13*, pp. 282–283. Copyright 1994 by The Guilford Press. Reprinted by permission.

Consistent with this reasoning, people's recollections of the feelings accompanying the two emotions were also substantially different. Embarrassed people felt awkward, but shameful people felt immoral and were more likely to consider themselves bad people. Embarrassing mistakes were "temporary errors," but shameful deficiencies were "deep-seated flaws." Embarrassment was short-lived and mild, whereas shame was stronger and lasted longer.

Finally, in keeping with these different types of transgressions, embarrassment seemed more surprising and accidental than shame. Shame developed more slowly and was often foreseen in some way. The behaviors that produce shame are evidently more voluntary and intentional than those that produce embarrassment (Manstead & Tetlock, 1989; Mosher & White, 1981).

Overall, then, our first attempt to delineate embarrassment and shame indicated that potentially reliable, meaningful differences did exist. Shame did appear to be a stronger, more enduring emotion that is more intense in part because of the more fearsome events with which it is associated: People are surprised and discombobulated by embarrassment, but they feel dissolute and deeply flawed in shame. Embarrassment was often remembered as a funny accident that was only bothersome because others knew about it; by comparison, shame was neither funny nor accidental, and could occur even in private if people learned unpleasant things about themselves that they would prefer not to know. In short, embarrassment and shame seemed to result from recognizably different situations and to cause distinct feelings discriminable by more than mere intensity.

However, there was a potentially important limitation of our procedure in this first study; we pressed our participants to make fine distinctions between embarrassment and shame that may have exaggerated the differences between them. For example, although our participants felt that the presence of an audience characterized embarrassment better than shame, concern over others' evaluations may also play an important, though perhaps less central role, in shame. The sorting procedure we used did not allow us to assess the *extent* to which these descriptors fit one emotion better than another.

For that reason, June Tangney, Laura Flicker, Deborah Barlow, and I conducted a second study that asked participants to *rate* remembered shame and embarrassment episodes on dimensions suggested by our first investigation (Tangney et al., 1996). Again, respondents vividly recalled past experiences of shame and embarrassment, but on this occasion, they provided detailed ratings of the feelings and reactions associated with each emotion. We also compared embarrassment to guilt.

This more exacting procedure again suggested that shame (and guilt) were quite different from embarrassment. Almost a fifth (18%) of the remembered shame experiences occurred when no one else was present, but almost no (only 2%) embarrassments occurred when people were alone. When they occurred, both shame and guilt were more intense, more painful, and more lasting emotions that had more moral implications than embarrassment did. There were several other differences, however, that had nothing to do with the greater intensity and moral relevance of shame. Embarrassment occurred more suddenly, was more surprising, made people less angry, and was funnier. People felt less blameworthy and less sad when they were embarrassed, but they felt more exposed and conspicuous. They also reported stronger physical changes in embarrassment than in the other two emotions.

Altogether, our studies suggest that embarrassment is obviously distinct from shame. It emerges from different antecedent events, has a very different phenomenology, and even seems to be reflected in recognizably different facial expressions and behavior (see Chapter 8, and Keltner & Buswell, 1996). Both emotions require advanced human capacities for self-consciousness (Tangney & Fischer, 1995), and both emerge from unwanted predicaments, but they have little else in common. Shame is angry, hurtful, and divisive, whereas embarrassment is silly and rather useful; as we'll see in later chapters, embarrassment is a desirable emotion that serves valuable functions in social life. Shame motivates aggressive, self-serving behavior, and seems much less adaptive; it makes the guilty party feel badly, but can easily wound innocent parties, as well.

## CONCLUSIONS

We often laugh at past embarrassments, but there's nothing funny about shame, and that is just one of several important differences that make embarrassment and shame discrete, nonoverlapping emotions. They may not always seem to be different because any given emotional experience may be a combination or succession of different affects, all influenced by social context and carelessly inspected or understood. Moreover, to the extent that our emotion knowledge is based on overlapping prototypes with fuzzy boundaries, it may be more vague than we realize. As we experience them, many episodes of embarrassment and shame may seem more similar than different unless we go to the trouble to assess our feelings thoughtfully. Nevertheless, as we have seen, there *are* reliable distinctions between embarrassment and shame.

In fact, we should seriously consider the possibility that embarrassment is distinctive enough, with regard to its antecedents, physiology, and signals to be regarded as a basic emotion. I have only been able to introduce that argument in this chapter because there is much that bears on embarrassment's status as a basic emotion that I have yet to discuss in detail. Still, even at this juncture, it may be time to recognize that not only is embarrassment *not* just a weak form of shame, it can reasonably be said to be one of a small handful of central emotions that have played especially formative roles in shaping human experience. It is distinctive. More importantly, despite its often laughable aspects, it seems to have functions and uses that make it an indispensable ingredient of normal humanity. This is a daring assertion, but I think it is supportable, and I'll try to convince you of it in the chapters ahead.

# CHAPTER 3

# Embarrassing Circumstances

❧

The pervasive importance of embarrassment in daily life is reflected, in part, by the variety of incidents that can cause embarrassment. Diverse events can create sudden discombobulation and flustered chagrin, and the potential for embarrassment lurks within most public activities in an ordinary day. We may be simply crossing a street, as Marie was when her slip ensnared her feet, or chatting with a friend, as I was when I drenched a new acquaintance with a soft drink, when we inadvertently make unwanted mistakes. Or, our conduct may be exemplary; we may behave impeccably but still be singled out for razzing and teasing by others who want to watch us squirm. Whenever we are in the company of others, unanticipated, undesired predicaments that threaten our social images are possible, and the threat of embarrassment exists.

In this and the next chapter, I'll provide a comprehensive catalogue of embarrassing circumstances. An attempt to organize embarrassing plights into meaningful categories is interesting in its own right; as we'll see, various kinds of hilarious and remarkable predicaments befall people all the time. There are more subtle advantages of an embarrassment catalogue as well. A survey of embarrassing predicaments allows us to test our knowledge of *why* embarrassment occurs. Useful explanations must flexibly encompass all the situations that cause embarrassment. These various circumstances also encourage other questions: How do we gradually come to dread these events? After all, very young children show little reaction to invasions of privacy (for instance) that would fluster adults. Further, do these events affect everyone the same way? Not everyone may respond similarly to a given predicament, and some people may be harder to embarrass than others. These issues of the origins of embarrassment, and differences among people in susceptibility to embarrassment, are important enough that we will consider them in detail in coming chapters. Nevertheless, they derive, in part, from the analysis of embarrassing circumstances we are about to conduct. Thus, our current focus: What events cause embarrassment?

## EARLY STUDIES

The very first empirical studies of embarrassment addressed this question. In 1964, Edward Gross and Gregory Stone collected hundreds of anecdotal accounts of embarrassment from college students and colleagues, and concluded that embarrassing incidents were generally of three types. In each, a central component of interaction is disrupted, leaving participants ill at ease and unsure of what to do or say next.

First, problems of inconsistent, mistaken, or unsupported *identity* can occur. For instance, people might fail to support their claims to a particular identity by finding that, after they have eaten a meal at a restaurant, they have left their wallets at home. Being unable to pay for the meal or prove who they are, they would risk the embarrassment of being thought to be undesirable characters. People might also misplay an identity, allowing incompatible information to intrude on the impressions they are attempting to create. For example, a young man trying to seem sophisticated at an opera might be embarrassed if his mispronunciation of the title "Die Fledermaus" reveals him to be a neophyte.[1] Finally, one could mistake people's identities, forgetting people's names or confusing them with others.

A second source of embarrassments is the loss of *poise*, the control of one's self or situation. Poor management of the tools of interaction such as (1) territory, as when one blunders into an occupied bathroom; (2) equipment, as when one's car stalls in a busy intersection; (3) clothes, as when one's pants rip; or even (4) one's body, as when one's stomach growls loudly, can all cause embarrassment.

Finally, Gross and Stone suggested that embarrassment can result from a loss of *confidence*, when a person's assumptions about others are shaken. Anyone interacting with someone else who loses poise or misplays an identity could find him- or herself in a confusing predicament; interactive surprises could leave one befuddled and unsure of how to proceed, and such awkward uncertainty could be embarrassing.

Thus, this first analysis of embarrassing circumstances suggested that embarrassment results from a variety of events that disrupt the smooth, predictable flow of social interaction. Partners in interaction were thought to adopt coherent, recognizable roles—patterns of behavior on which they and others could agree and depend—and whenever partners' expectations were violated, the flustered discomfort of embarrassment could result.

Interestingly, Gross and Stone further suggested that, whereas most embarrassments were unexpected and undesired, some episodes were deliberately caused by others. On occasion, people were singled out and embarrassed on purpose by other people using such tactics as "practical jokes, teasing, initiation into secret societies, puncturing false fronts, and public degradation" (Gross & Stone, 1964, p. 13). Despite the fact that such treatment could cause the victim considerable chagrin, deliberate embarrassment was presumed to be enacted by others for various reasons. First, it could be used as punishment for undesirable behavior. Violations of social norms might be met with corrective derision from one's peers that would serve to point out one's mistakes. Embarrassment could thus be used as a tool of socialization with which youngsters could be taught appropriate conduct (an important point we will examine further in Chapter 5). In addition, deliberate embarrassments could be employed strategically to establish and maintain social power. Anyone claiming an undeserved status within a social group could be targeted for embarrassment, which would, for instance, "put her in her place."

As we will see, this analysis overlooked many subtle types of embarrassment. In particular, more recent investigations suggest that deliberate embarrassment is used as often to establish friendly solidarity with others (e.g., in innocuous, friendly teasing) as to bring a braggart down a notch (Sharkey, 1992, 1993). Nevertheless, Gross and Stone's first foray established that embarrassment could be caused either by personal misbehavior or by the intentional or unintentional actions of others. It also suggested that social interaction was so complex, there were various ways it could go wrong with embarrassing results.

In a subsequent paper, Martin Weinberg (1968) acknowledged the embarrassing potential of losses of identity, poise, or confidence, but he asserted that two more fundamental dimensions underlay such events. He suggested that behavior that becomes embarrassing could be either intended or unintended, and based on either a correct or an incorrect definition of the situation. Together, the two dimensions described four elementary forms of embarrassment: faux pas, accidents, mistakes, and duties.

The first of these, *faux pas*, occurs when one's intentional behavior later turns out to have been based on an inaccurate assessment of the situation. In one such case, actor David Niven once arrived in clown's makeup for a Halloween party that turned out to be formal black tie (Morley, 1983). (He says he was never invited back.) On other occasions, one's expectations may be correct, but one's behavior unintended;

these are *accidents*, such as spilling coffee in one's lap. Incorrect definitions of a situation can also lead to unintended actions that are *mistakes*.
A male professor who wrongly believes that his pants zipper is closed
when he steps before a class would be making a mistake. Finally,
Weinberg suggested that even intended behavior and correct definitions
could cause embarrassment when one performed unwanted *duties*, such
as a young girl submitting to her first gynecological examination.

This last type is an interesting category. One can readily imagine
the unease with which an adolescent first allows a heretofore forbidden
activity, the deliberate inspection of her genitalia by a mere acquaintance. One can further imagine the awkwardness with which a young
adult medical student may first conduct such a consultation. In both
cases, the embarrassed person is behaving appropriately and is doing
nothing that would make a negative impression on others. On the other
hand, in both cases the embarrassed person is engaging in an unfamiliar
action that, in different contexts, *would* be inappropriate; a new, unprac-
ticed "identity" is being tried, with behavior that transcends old norms
of conduct. According to Weinberg, such legitimate activities engender
embarrassment through one's personal sense that an old rule is being
broken, even if others don't seem to care. These two observations—first,
that embarrassment can occur in the absence of any overt mistake or
predicament, and second, that embarrassment does not require the
censure of outside observers—are potentially important points to which
we will return.

A third analysis of embarrassment was provided by Jerome Sattler
in 1965. In an ambitious project, Sattler asked 301 people, including
eighth-graders, college students, institutionalized schizophrenics, and
normal adults in their 30s, to list up to 20 situations they considered
embarrassing. More than 3,000 embarrassing events were obtained, and,
with the exception of a few bizarre examples provided by the schizophrenics (e.g., "I am embarrassed when I stand close to fire" [p. 31]),
they generally fit the categories described thus far. Failures of propriety,
privacy, competency, and grace were routine, and common to all four
groups of participants. However, there were several discoveries in the
data that were new contributions.

First, Sattler organized the incidents by noting that people were
often the *agents* of their own embarrassment, becoming embarrassed
when their own actions caused them chagrin. Such incidents included
those identified by Weinberg (1968) and the failures of identity or poise
noted by Gross and Stone (1964). In other cases, people became embarrassed when they were the *recipients* or targets of others' actions; just as
Gross and Stone had found, people were often embarrassed when others
teased or criticized them. Remarkably, people also reported that they

could be embarrassed by receiving too much praise. One college male wrote, "I feel embarrassed when someone says good things about me" (Sattler, 1965, p. 31). Such accounts were intriguing, because, with the possible exception of the uncomfortable duties described by Weinberg (1968), other embarrassments all seemed to fit a general model of obvious public miscues or disruption. The suggestion that others could embarrass us by being too complimentary was one of several new types of embarrassment Sattler observed.

Another such type was simple conspicuousness, in which (either as agent or recipient) a person became the center of attention of a group of people. Curiously, feeling singled out for inspection by others was often embarrassing even when there was nothing deficient or untoward about one's behavior. As one example, an adult female reported that "it is embarrassing to walk into a roomful of people and have them look at me such as at my first PTA meeting" (Sattler, 1965, p. 31). Evidently, scattered among the thousands of embarrassing events listed by Sattler's respondents were subtle circumstances that did not easily fit the compact schemes of other researchers.

A third broad category of embarrassments was new as well. Sattler found that people could be mere *observers* of others' actions but be embarrassed by them nonetheless. Simply witnessing another person's embarrassing predicament was sometimes enough to cause personal discomfort, even when one was just a bystander. The embarrassed target could be a relative or friend well known to the observer (e.g., "I am embarrassed when my wife is embarrassed" [Sattler, 1965, p. 33]), or just a stranger (e.g., "I am embarrassed if I see someone else go through an embarrassing experience" [p. 33]), but in either case, observer embarrassment was possible.

Sattler's work thus took the study of embarrassing circumstances beyond the obvious incidents of personal blunder and mishap that most readily come to mind as embarrassing. By encouraging (and sometimes nagging) his respondents to think of several different events they had found embarrassing, Sattler demonstrated that people were occasionally discombobulated by incidents that did not necessarily endanger their identities or interactions at all. Being an innocent center of attention, receiving acclaim, or just witnessing others' predicaments might all embarrass at least some of the people some of the time.

## EXPERIMENTAL INVESTIGATIONS

Years later, the three surveys of the 1960s were the foundation for two experimental studies of embarrassment by younger researchers. In both cases, investigators sought to determine whether relatively subtle forms of embarrassment reported by Sattler's (1965) respondents really did exist.

## Overpraise

In the first of these, Laura Buss (1978) examined the impact of excessive praise, or "overpraise." College men and women first rated their attractiveness and interpersonal sensitivity, and then, weeks later, as part of an ostensible study of "first impressions," received face-to-face evaluations from an experimental assistant they had just met. All four combinations of male and female evaluators and targets were tried, and three kinds of evaluation were provided. In a control condition, the evaluators gave feedback that matched what the subjects had earlier said about themselves. In an "underpraise" condition, subjects received poorer evaluations than they felt they deserved. However, the remaining participants received glowing praise that exceeded their self-evaluations, and thus encountered "overpraise." Blushing and other signs of embarrassment were observed in nearly all the subjects who received excessive compliments, but occurred rarely in those who received their due, or less. Overpraise appeared to produce embarrassment, as Buss predicted it would.

## Empathic Embarrassment

Another investigation was my first study of embarrassment (Miller, 1987). I believed that "empathic embarrassment" was possible, and that, just as Sattler's respondents had reported, people could be embarrassed by witnessing others' social predicaments.[2] I distinguished empathic embarrassment from the personal embarrassment that occurs when our associates transgress and we are appropriately concerned with what third-party audiences think of us (as any parent may be embarrassed by a child's tantrum in a crowded grocery store). True empathic embarrassment would occur, I believed, only if people became embarrassed by observing a stranger's public predicament in a situation in which the stranger's plight did not bear on the observers' own social identities at all.

To study such a possibility, I asked pairs of college students who did not know each other, either two men or two women, to report to my lab at the University of Florida. There, they either cooperated on a brief task, competed against each other, or, in a third condition, completed the task separately, maintaining total independence from one another. Afterwards, a flip of a coin assigned each of them to an *actor* or *observer* role. The observer was then taken to an adjacent room where he or she could clearly see the actor through a one-way observation window without being seen in return. There, one of two possible sets of instructions awaited the observer, who was asked either to watch the actor's behavior carefully, noting "hand gestures" and "shifts in body carriage," or, instead, to try to imagine what the actor was feeling, visualizing how it feels to be performing the tasks. These latter instructions were adapted from prior studies of empathy (e.g., Gould & Sigall, 1977), and were meant to direct observers' attention to any embarrassment the actors might feel.

Next door, each actor was asked to perform either *embarrassing* or *innocuous* tasks. The luck of the draw determined what happened; the actor blindly picked a sheet of instructions from an envelope that contained both sets of tasks. Half of the actors were instructed to (1) sing "The Star Spangled Banner," using the available sheet music if they wished; (2) laugh for 30 seconds as if they had just heard a joke; (3) start a tape player and dance to the recorded pop music for 60 seconds; and finally, (4) to imitate a 5-year-old throwing a temper tantrum because he or she did not want to go to bed. Obviously, these were the embarrassing tasks, invented and shown to be effective by Robert Apsler (1975, in a study we'll describe in Chapter 9). "The Star Spangled Banner" spans a full octave, so that it's typical for people's voices to crack on the highest notes (i.e., "the rocket's red glare"). Chuckling to oneself is easy for the first 5 seconds or so, but quickly becomes awkward and strained over a longer period. (Try it as you read this, and see for yourself.) Many of us may dance alone when we're vacuuming or folding laundry, but not when others are watching! In each case, the embarrassing tasks were *meant* to cause some chagrin and abashment, especially compared to the nonembarrassing tasks, which were mild indeed. An actor drawing the innocuous tasks was simply asked to *listen* to the recorded music and to *write* down the words of "The Star Spangled Banner," among other tasks.

Finally, the actor was left alone to perform the tasks as the observer watched. The primary question, of course, involved the observers: Was empathic embarrassment possible? While they were watching the actors, the electrical conductivity of the observers' skin was measured via electrodes attached to a hand and arm; this procedure assessed the small changes in the skin that are indicative of emotional arousal. Afterwards, the observers reported their perceptions of the actors and described their own feelings during the tasks.

In general, both the actors and observers were more affected by the embarrassing than the innocuous tasks. The actors found the former tasks to be much more embarrassing, and the observers found them more compelling to watch, especially when they were asked to concentrate on the actors' feelings. Interestingly, the observers reported stronger reactions of various types; they were sorry for the embarrassed actors, but also reported greater enjoyment of their tasks. However, the observers also said it embarrassed them to watch the actors' exotic performances, and their physical measures of emotional arousal were more highly related to these self-reports of embarrassment than to any other emotion. The observers apparently encountered a mixture of feelings watching the spectacles next door, but part of their responses involved aversive arousal that could reasonably be called empathic embarrassment.

Lower levels of empathic embarrassment were felt by the observers when they were instructed to watch body movements dispassionately instead of thinking about the actors' feelings. Further, less empathic embarrassment occurred when the observers had had no prior contact with the actors, instead of cooperating or competing with them previously. Nevertheless, it was clear that onlookers could be affected by the embarrassing predicaments of total strangers and that empathic embarrassment was possible.

Remember, this was not an especially new idea. Sattler's (1965) respondents had reported such occurrences, and Erving Goffman had also argued that "when an individual finds himself in a situation which ought to make him blush, others present usually will blush with him" (1956, p. 265). Some of the people who participated in my study (Miller, 1987) even volunteered their own accounts of empathic embarrassment during the question-and-answer period that followed their participation. For instance, some had been pained by reruns of episodes of "I Love Lucy" on television; Lucy got herself into such predicaments that young adults would actually change channels to avoid her fictional plights![3] What was new about my study was the effort to elicit such a subtle phenomenon under controlled conditions in a lab. Because (1) this is one of the first experimental studies we have described in detail, and (2) I was personally involved, I'd like to say a few more things about it.

### Embarrassment in the Laboratory

The good news about embarrassment research is that it is one of the few emotions, positive or negative, that can be quickly produced, in full flower, through laboratory manipulations. Positive or negative moods can be induced with various ploys; listening to slow, funereal music can make people glum (Wenzlaff, Wegner, & Klein, 1991) and winning an unexpected $2.00 cash prize can brighten their moods (Mackie & Worth, 1989). Emotions are harder to study, either because events that are under experimental control cannot produce them or because researchers would be reluctant to do so. Consider anger, sadness, and joy; although they are open to experimentation, it is difficult to influence events that matter enough to people to produce full-fledged experiences of these emotions. Different concerns confront studies of fear or shame; whereas people can be scared or induced to do shameful things, researchers may not wish to create robust experiences of these emotions— for instance, to temporarily terrify their subjects—out of concern for the well-being of the research participants.

Embarrassment *can* be readily created in an experiment, with participants randomly assigned to conditions that will or will not embarrass them. Apsler (1975) devised the four silly tasks described above; a variety of other procedures, ranging from sucking a baby's pacifier (Brown, 1970) to staged accidents (Gonzales, Pederson, Manning, & Wetter, 1990) and physical measurement of one's body fat (Leary, Rejeski, et al., 1994) have been employed successfully. The bad news is that nobody likes to be embarrassed, and it's true that subjects in embarrassment studies may encounter temporary discomfort. However, laboratory embarrassments are moderate and brief enough that they can be safely implemented without any lasting harm or undue stress to the participants. No procedure used by a reputable researcher creates reactions stronger than the ordinary experiences people might routinely encounter outside the lab. Moreover, participants can always decline to continue, or not to begin at all, if they feel too much chagrin. Participants are always volunteers who have acknowledged in writing their right to quit a study at any time. Most importantly, embarrassment research is not conducted frivolously. A serious academic purpose always underlies researchers' attempts to make people embarrassed.

Admittedly, these remarks are completely unnecessary for most readers of this book, who are familiar with the practice and ethics of psychological research. Still, some readers may be wondering whether it was really reasonable for me to ask people to do things that I knew would be embarrassing. I think it was. No one had to do them, and in fact 3% of my participants chose to quit when they read the list of tasks. They were graciously excused without any sort of penalty. Those who did continue were ultimately provided with a complete explanation of the purpose, design, and intent of the study; their criticisms were solicited, and they were heartily thanked. And, as you might expect, most seemed to enjoy the experience. The study was, after all, fairly entertaining, and the discussions that followed the procedure were usually lively and always amicable.

My point is that embarrassment is amenable to manageable and sensitive experimental inquiry. Studies of embarrassment employ reasonable procedures that create real emotion without lasting harm.

Moreover, they are worth doing. Ideally, this book demonstrates that individual studies provide cumulative insights that gradually produce meaningful understanding, and that understanding of embarrassment is our goal.

## EMBARRASSMENT'S SOCIAL SITUATIONS

I've shown that a variety of different, sometimes subtle events can cause embarrassment, and I am almost in position to describe a comprehensive catalogue of embarrassing circumstances. There are still some general points to make, however. A few studies have shed light on the social contexts in which embarrassment is most likely to occur, and I should note that a given event may or may not cause embarrassment depending on whether or not anyone else is present and (if others are present) who those others are.

### Can We Be Embarrassed When We're Alone?

As we saw in Chapter 1, embarrassment usually involves a sense of exposure and conspicuousness, coupled with an awkward concern for what others are thinking of us. These characteristics obviously depend on the belief that others are aware of our miscues, and embarrassment may thus be stronger as we become increasingly certain that others (1) do know of our misbehavior and (2) do think we're inept. On the other hand, these characteristics also suggest that if we are sure that our actions are private, we may be immune to embarrassment. Accidents or mistakes that would unquestionably be embarrassing in public may lose their impact if we are convinced that no one else knows about them. Folk wisdom, as proffered by the popular comic strip character "Garfield" the cat, suggests just such a view. Envision this "Garfield" strip: Ensnared in a window blind, dangling high off the floor, Garfield thinks to himself, "I'd cry out for help, but I couldn't handle that; predicaments are embarrassing only when noticed by someone else" (Davis, 1981, p. 6B).

Certainly, some events lose their effect if no one else knows about them. Consider the losses of poise described by Gross and Stone (1964): Splitting one's pants is likely to be embarrassing at a party, but not on a solitary backpacking trip. Similarly, a bout of loud hiccuping may be amusing in the shower but embarrassing at a lecture. In these and many other cases, particular events lose their embarrassing potential if they cannot endanger one's social identity by becoming known to others.

Nevertheless, not all of the embarrassments people encounter are public events. I and my colleagues have now conducted three large surveys of embarrassing incidents, collecting hundreds of accounts of past or present embarrassments in each investigation (Miller, 1992; Stonehouse & Miller, 1994; Tangney et al., 1996).[4] The vast majority of predicaments that cause embarrassment, 98% or higher in each sample, are public. However, there are always some accounts of embarrassments that have occurred even when no one but the hapless victim is aware of them.

Here's an example. A female college student wrote:

> "I was waiting to take a Spanish test, so I decided to go and use the bathroom. I walked in and was looking in the mirror when I noticed a strange urinal behind me! I realized that I was in the men's restroom. Luckily, no one saw me! But I was still very embarrassed."

In another instance a fifth grader disclosed, "I tripped over the clothes basket. No one was around." These cases appear to involve genuinely private events that were nevertheless embarrassing. Public exposure is a component of prototypical embarrassment (Parrott & Smith, 1991), but it is evidently not required for some forms of embarrassment to occur.

We may need to take account of two factors here. First, through simple repetition, the chagrin and abashment we experience after public mishaps may gradually generalize to any private events that resemble them. If (and I am making up this example!) a professor is famous for—and humiliated by—appearing before his class at least once a month with his pants zipper open, he may experience weaker but similar chagrin when he discovers himself unzipped on his private drive to work. A public predicament has been averted, but the close parallel between the public and private events is likely to elicit a moment of similar emotion. Relatively automatic processes of classical conditioning would predict such outcomes and make weak forms of "private embarrassment" possible.

More interesting are a person's own conceptions of his or her private acts. More than a century ago, Charles Darwin suggested that people might blush in private when they consider "what others would have thought . . . had they known of the act" (1872/1965, p. 335). Recall that Weinberg (1968) also proposed that people could be embarrassed by "duties" they found distasteful even if no external audience would consider them in the wrong. Perhaps a person's own negative evaluations of the social appropriateness of his or her behavior can cause embarrassment, even when that behavior is private.

Andre Modigliani (1971) held such a view when he conducted an experiment in which, by chance, some participants publicly failed their portion of a group task, while others failed privately, and still others privately succeeded. Modigliani found that those whose failures were unknown to the group were less embarrassed than those who had publicly bungled their assignments, but more embarrassed than those who had not failed at all. Modigliani felt this result was due to a mild embarrassment that often exists in the absence of an audience, contending that "private-failure subjects allowed their sense of self-deficiency to produce an imagined sense of social disapproval" (p. 22). When we have misbehaved somehow, sitting and pondering, "What would they think? If they only knew . . ." may be enough to cause embarrassment (Miller, 1986).

On the other hand, such thoughts may not readily occur when a person is truly, completely alone. In Modigliani's (1971) study, the private failure participants believed that some of their subsequent performances would be public, so the prospect of social evaluation loomed large. Similarly, when the college student found herself in the men's restroom, she faced the threat of mortifying discovery at any moment. These events were private, but the potential for social disapproval was real. In the same way, a solitary hiker may be embarrassed by split pants if he or she has no change of clothes, and must dread the slow return to civilization.

Thus private embarrassment appears to be possible, but such episodes usually involve conscious (if passing) recognition of what others would think if one's behavior were more widely known. When the threat of discovery is real, such episodes don't *feel* private, and an embarrassed person is likely to be as focused on others' potential evaluations as is a victim of a more public predicament. This is probably also true when one engages in unfamiliar, personally undesirable public behavior—Weinberg's (1968) "duties"—in the absence of overt disdain. On those other occasions when one is certain of privacy, private embarrassment may occur but is unlikely, because one is less apt to vividly envision the social disapproval that normally produces embarrassment. As Barry Schlenker asserted, "social predicaments do exist in 'private' . . . all that is required is *an imagined audience that prompts attention to the self as a social object*" (1980, p. 130). If a person hasn't the time or motivation to reflect on what would happen "if they only knew," private embarrassment should not occur. Garfield the cat's folk wisdom should be revised to note that "predicaments are embarrassing only when we vividly imagine them being noticed by someone else."

Finally, we should note that a process like this may also occur when we don't recognize a public predicament until after it's over. People may be alone when they discover that a past predicament took place, but still become embarrassed when they envision the situation they *were* in. In one such case, a college student was embarrassed when he feel asleep in an afternoon class and woke up to find the classroom deserted (Miller, 1992). As far as he knows, no one noticed him as the class ended and everyone departed, but he thought it more likely that he had been conspicuous and laughable, and he was embarrassed even though he was presently alone. Our conceptualizations of events can embarrass us, even when no audience is present at the time.

## The Number of Onlookers

In any case, private embarrassment is rare; only about 1 out of every 50 embarrassments occurs when no one else is around. In contrast, other emotions such as shame and guilt are much more likely to occur privately; 1 of every 10 experiences of guilt and almost 1 of every 5 episodes of shame occur with no one else present (Tangney et al., 1996). As we saw in Chapter 2, embarrassment normally involves more single-minded attention to others' evaluations of oneself than shame and guilt do; one's social image is usually of more central concern in embarrassment than in the other two emotions. It should be no surprise, therefore, that embarrassment is a more public emotion that is less likely to occur under private conditions.

Furthermore, embarrassment ordinarily occurs in front of larger audiences. The mistakes and accidents that cause embarrassment may occur anytime, even in front of fairly large groups of strangers. For instance, a respondent in one of my studies—who described slipping down onto her buttocks with her arms full of groceries in front of the grocery store—counted eight people who witnessed her embarrassing spill. In comparison, the more momentous transgressions that underlie shame and guilt are likely to emerge from more meaningful interactions with others that involve fewer numbers of people. Thus, when we obtained detailed narratives of emotional experiences from adult respondents, we found that nearly seven other people were present, on average, when embarrassment occurred. In contrast, only three others were usually present when people felt shame or guilt (Tangney et al., 1996).

The bigger the audience, the stronger one's embarrassment is likely to be. When I dumped that large soft drink on the head of a new acquaintance (back in Chapter 1), I would have been embarrassed if only she and I were present. I was more embarrassed because her husband was there too, and it was even worse that I soaked her during the busy lunch hour at a campus cafeteria with dozens of others about. (It was quite the public spectacle.) The greater the number of onlookers, the more widespread the potential damage to one's social identity, and the more intense one's resultant embarrassment will usually be.

Don Shearn and his colleagues documented this effect when they examined blushing and skin conductance responses in students at Colorado College (Shearn, Bergman, Hill, Abel, & Hinds, 1992). First, they prepared videotapes of women singing "The Star Spangled Banner." Then, a day later, either one or four other people were present as the women watched either their own embarrassing performances or (in order to create a different kind of aversive emotion) the notorious shower murder scene from the movie *Psycho*. They blushed when watching themselves, but not when watching *Psycho*, and they blushed more intensely when the larger audience was present than when only one other person watched them sing. The other measures of physiological arousal behaved similarly, and the women clearly seemed more embarrassed when more witnesses were present.

Interestingly, however, a professor who finds his zipper open in front of a class of 500 students will probably be only slightly more abashed than he would have been with a smaller class of 50. Adding more and more witnesses to a person's predicament probably increases that person's embarrassment by smaller and smaller amounts. Bibb Latané's (1981) Social Impact Theory predicts that there is "a marginally decreasing effect" (p. 344) on our emotions of each new person that is added to an evaluative audience. The difference between an audience of 14 or 15 people, for instance, is presumed to be much smaller than the difference between an audience of only one person and an audience of two. Latané and Harkins (1976) supported this prediction by asking people to estimate how much stage fright they would experience with audiences of varying sizes, and Latané (1981) reports a variety of findings from diverse investigations that are all consistent with the Social Impact Theory. It is reasonable to assume, then, that once a sizable crowd is present—and a person is quite mortified—a much bigger audience is likely to increase that person's embarrassment only slightly.

### The Nature of the Audience

Some of the events we encounter make us look so foolish or inept that having *anyone* else around would be embarrassing. Nevertheless, the amount of embarrassment that results from a predicament—and, perhaps, whether embarrassment occurs at all—may depend on exactly who else is present. Consider a father on a fishing trip with his teenaged sons who, while relaxing around the campfire at the end of the day, inadvertently emits an unmistakably audible and aromatic bit of intestinal gas. If his sons are elsewhere, upwind, he is unlikely to be embarrassed by his private act. However, even if his sons are there, he may be only mildly abashed; they may think his behavior crude, but he can reasonably count on their forbearance and quick forgiveness. Now, contrast that outcome with the intense mortification that might result if a similar event occurred at a business meeting or on a blind date.

To the extent embarrassment is based on fear of negative evaluations from others, it should be less likely to occur when we are assured of others' lasting acceptance and approval. Day to day, we are certainly less concerned with impressing those who already know and like us. In a remarkable investigation, Mark Leary and John Nezlek obtained detailed records of all the important social interactions 179 Wake Forest University students encountered during a week's time (Leary, Nezlek, et al., 1994). After each interaction, the students described the other people with whom they had talked and reported the impressions they had wanted to make. In general, these young adults cared less about what their close, same-sex friends thought of them than they did about the impressions they made (1) on same-sex people they did not know well or (2) on anyone of the opposite sex. Among familiar friends, people let down their guard and were less interested in carefully regulating the impressions they made during a conversation.

On the one hand, this is a surprising result. People tried harder to influence the judgments of mere acquaintances than they did the evaluations of important friends. Because friends are more dear to us, a friend's acceptance and approval should be more valuable than similar regard from a casual acquaintance. On the other hand, Leary, Nezlek, et al.'s results are straightforward if we assume that people are especially relaxed around their same-sex friends because they can be confident that their friends hold them in high esteem. A friend's judgments do matter more, but we can usually count on friends' approbation; from moment to moment, people may be more concerned with eliciting liking from those whose approval is less certain (Jellison & Gentry, 1978), even if their relationships with those people are more superficial and less important.

In any case, some events that would cause embarrassment among acquaintances or strangers are less compelling if they happen among friends (see Froming, Corley, & Rinker, 1990). I'm aware of a reasonably dramatic example that makes this very point. While in graduate school, a friend of mine visited a popular bar for "Quarter Time," a happy-hour promotion in which cocktails went on sale for $0.25 apiece and went up a quarter in price every 15 minutes. This was a particularly unhealthy idea, as it encouraged poor but crafty students to drink as quickly as possible to get the most for their money. In any case, my friend drank too much, too fast, and ultimately became ill. When he was out in his companion's car in the parking lot, he threw open the door, leaned out, and vomited on the pavement. Being with a good friend (and being drunk), he recalls only mild chagrin until, with the last heaves leaving him, he picked up his head and saw, just inches away, a woman's shoes. He had had a wider audience than he initially believed; two women had just climbed out of their adjacent car when he threw open his door and vomited at their feet. *That's* when he really became embarrassed.

Linda MacDonald and Martin Davies (1983) provided a more scientific demonstration of this point when they embarrassed college students by involving them in an awkward conversation with an experimental accomplice. Watching from another room was either a stranger or a same-sex friend of the embarrassed student. When the accomplice accused the hapless students of asking prying, personal questions, they actually became more embarrassed when they didn't know the person witnessing the event than when a reliable friend was watching. Undoubtedly, the strangers were the less influential critics, but the participants probably felt at greater risk of receiving threatening social disapproval from the strangers than the friends. In general, embarrassment is probably less likely or less intense when we can be sure of continued regard from those who witness it.

June Tangney and I corroborated this conclusion by asking respondents to describe the audiences that were present when they became embarrassed (Tangney et al., 1996). Embarrassment was significantly less likely to occur among loved ones and much more likely to occur among strangers and acquaintances than were shame and guilt. In addition, all three emotions rarely occurred when subordinates of lower prestige and power were present. (This result may be due to the rarity with which the respondents, who were college students, actually found themselves among subordinates. Nevertheless, it is consistent with the idea that embarrassment is unlikely when we can afford not to care what an audience thinks of us.)

Audiences of high status and prestige may be especially threatening and may cause stronger embarrassment if a predicament develops (Latané, 1981; Leary & Kowalski, 1990). Curiously, however, a mixed audience of both high and low prestige observers may actually cause less embarrassment than a *smaller* audience containing only those of high prestige. Catherine and John Seta (1992) have shown that the stage fright created by a particular audience depends on two characteristics of the observers. First, the *total* size and status of the audience are influential, so that, as we have seen, larger crowds are more threatening and more prestigious audiences are more intimidating. In addition, however, the *average* composition of an audience impels our emotions, so that a larger audience with lower average prestige may be less unsettling than a smaller group of higher status. Seta and Seta (1992) ingeniously demonstrated this effect by measuring the blood pressure of college students who performed for an "audience" made up of (1) a professor, (2) a high school student, (3) two high school students, or (4) both the professor and a student. Adding a second student when one was already present made the performers more anxious, increasing their blood pressure; average prestige remained constant, but the total size of the audience went up. Remarkably, adding the same student to the audience containing the professor actually reduced the performers' anxiety; the audience got bigger but its average prestige went down, and the averaging effect was apparently the more important influence. Seta and Seta have not yet specifically studied embarrassment, but their studies of related emotions reasonably suggest that averaging effects pertain there, too. The amount of embarrassment we feel probably depends on the overall, average nature of an audience as well as its total size and stature.

## CONCLUSIONS

The surveys of the 1960s established that embarrassment may follow diverse events. Thereafter, occasional laboratory investigations elicited reactions such as empathic embarrassment, demonstrated the dangers of overpraise, and showed that an audience of strangers could be more fearsome than an audience of friends. Obviously, depending on who is present at the time, a broad array of incidents may cause embarrassment.

Only recently, however, have researchers used the accumulated literature on embarrassment to construct an encyclopedic catalogue of embarrassing predicaments. Several studies in the 1990s have now contributed to a comprehensive description of the sources of embarrassment, which provides a useful foundation for ongoing research. Such a catalogue will be valuable to our further understanding of embarrassment as well, so I'll examine it in detail in the next chapter.

# CHAPTER 4

# A Catalogue
# of Embarrassments

∽

There have been three developmental stages in the scientific study of embarrassment. The sociologist Erving Goffman broke ground in 1956 with a theoretical framework that treated embarrassment as a disruption of the normal processes of social interaction. His intriguing approach (which we will treat in detail in Chapter 7) made embarrassment a respectable field of inquiry, and provided the impetus for the first empirical studies of embarrassment in the 1960s and early 1970s. Among these were the early surveys of embarrassment's circumstances by Gross and Stone (1964), Sattler (1965), and Weinberg (1968), and laboratory experiments such as those we've mentioned by Modigliani (1971) and Brown (1970). Thereafter, in its adolescence, embarrassment research gradually gained steam and became more diverse as the interactive consequences of social predicaments began to be studied (e.g., Apsler, 1975; Semin & Manstead, 1981). Occasional investigations focused on subtle or exotic forms of embarrassment such as overpraise (L. Buss, 1978) and empathic embarrassment (Miller, 1987), as well.

The current mature phase of inquiry into the nature and processes of embarrassment began, I think, with the publication in 1987 of the first monograph on embarrassment, by Robert Edelmann. This wide-ranging, integrative work demonstrated that embarrassment studies had reached critical mass; they constituted an eclectic but recognizably coherent field of inquiry complete with theoretical controversy, scholars who identified themselves with the field, and fascinating findings of some importance. Since Edelmann's book, embarrassment research has drifted toward the mainstream of social science as scholars have realized how well the embarrassing pitfalls of daily life can illuminate the motives and mechanics of normal interaction.

Nevertheless, the field reached this stage without ever completing the work begun by the analyses of embarrassing circumstances in the 1960s. Each of those studies was necessarily incomplete because each described embarrassments not encompassed by the others. And afterwards, save for conceptual work by Arnold Buss (1980), two decades passed without further effort to categorize the variety of events that can cause embarrassment.

Thus it was timely, if not a bit overdue, when two different research teams embarked in the early 1990s on efforts to create comprehensive catalogues of embarrassing circumstances. As we noted last chapter, such investigations offer a proving ground for our understanding of embarrassment. Moreover, because they involve the collection and synthesis of the remarkable predicaments that befall people, they are also a lot of fun.

## EMBARRASSING CIRCUMSTANCES REDUX

In one of these efforts, I asked people about the last time they were embarrassed (Miller, 1992). I had the opportunity to collect such accounts from students at Cornell University (in the state of New York), Wake Forest University (in North Carolina), and Sam Houston State University (in Texas); most of the participants were bona fide college students, but groups of high school students attending summer programs at Cornell and Sam Houston State also took part. Altogether, 350 people were asked to describe anonymously and in detail their most recent embarrassments, whether strong or weak. They were specifically asked not to recount their most dramatic or memorable predicaments, but to report their latest experiences of any embarrassment.

With rare exceptions, including one male collegian who wrote, "I have never been embarrassed," they were able to provide such accounts effortlessly. That was the easy part. Next, I and my colleagues Janet Duffy and Lee Ertsman had to make sense of the dizzying range of narratives. The good news was that we had the prior work of Gross and Stone (1964), Sattler (1965), and Weinberg (1968) to guide us; the bad news was that we were trying to expand on their work and produce a broader scheme than any of them had. We resorted to a method of analytic induction (Bulmer, 1979) that entailed the development of categories from a portion of the data, followed by a test of the emerging classifications with another portion of data. After two iterations, we had a set of 12 different categories of embarrassment that we could use reliably.

The individual categories seemed to show that embarrassing events were of four broad types. First, most predicaments resulted from *individual behavior* that was clumsy, forgetful, or hapless. In these events, a person autonomously created his or her own social dilemmas by tripping, misspeaking, belching, and so forth in public. In Sattler's (1965) terminology, these predicaments occurred when people were the agents of their own embarrassment, and the events encompassed all the situations described by Weinberg (1968) and the failures of identity and losses of poise identified by Gross and Stone (1964). Some of the events involved other people—for instance, forgetting an old acquaintance's name at a party—but these were generally misbehaviors one could also stumble into all on one's own.

In contrast, the three remaining types of embarrassment all entailed interaction with or intervention from other people. *Interactive* predicaments emerged from transactions with others in which a person and a particular partner (or partners) together produced embarrassing events for which the embarrassed person was not to blame. Such experiences were typically generated by incidents beyond the autonomous control of the embarrassed person and usually depended on the presence of particular interactive partners; that is, had different people been present, embarrassment would not have occurred. In such cases, the appropriate focus was not just the individual person who was embarrassed—who was blameless, after all—but the combination of that person and his or her social context; hence, the label "interactive" embarrassments.

In other situations, the fitting focus was squarely on the other people who either intentionally or unintentionally caused someone to become embarrassed. These were instances of *audience provocation* in which embarrassment would not have occurred without others' intervention. This type of embarrassment included those cases described by Sattler (1965) in which people were the unwitting recipients of embarrassment induced by others, and ranged from instances of people being deliberately singled out for brutal teasing to accidental dilemmas caused by a friend's inadvertent disclosures. In such situations, others' actions were always the present cause of a particular person's embarrassment.

Finally, people were occasionally embarrassed by being *bystanders* to others' predicaments. Merely witnessing someone else's embarrassing behavior could cause those watching to feel some uncomfortable chagrin of their own. In cases in which the observers had no obvious connection to the embarrassed person (so that their own public images were unaffected by the person's transgression), these were instances of empathic embarrassment (Miller, 1987), and Sattler's (1965) "observer" category fit here.

These four broad types of embarrassment encompassed the disparate categories of the earlier surveys of the 1960s, and had the advantage of implicitly suggesting an important dimension of embarrassing circumstances: Social predicaments ranged from events for which individuals were solely responsible to more interactive incidents in which the embarrassed victims played increasingly passive parts. However, the 12 specific categories of embarrassments we created were evidently incomplete; at the same time we were doing our survey, Bill Cupach and Sandra Metts of Illinois State University (1990, 1992; Metts & Cupach, 1989) were developing an impressive coding scheme of their own that included some predicaments that we had not identified.

Cupach and Metts also amassed recollections of embarrassment from college students and organized them into a coherent scheme. They grouped the accounts into only two broad types, those for which an embarrassed person was personally responsible and those for which other people were responsible. By doing so, I think they missed that intermediate class of embarrassments, the "interactive" predicaments, that aren't *anybody's* fault, resulting as they do from the unique combination of certain people with particular partners. However, Cupach and Metts did explicate a useful distinction among the embarrassments that are caused by others. In some cases, an embarrassed person is *directly involved* in the embarrassing episode because he or she is the specific target of the others' actions; someone who is teased by others is an intended victim, and thus is directly involved. In other instances, the embarrassed party is only *indirectly involved*, being the passive observer of actions that are not targeted personally at him or her; empathic embarrassment is a prime example. This distinction between direct and indirect involvement was implicit in the difference between my "audience provocation" and "bystander" categories, but Cupach and Metts were right to spell it out.

Their results also suggested several valuable refinements of the categories I had created. They subdivided audience provocations into specific acts such as teasing, criticism, recognition and praise, and violations of privacy and trust. Because such events may vary considerably with regard to whether they are actually intended to cause embarrassment, these were worthwhile distinctions. Cupach and Metts also described an intriguing category of embarrassment that I had missed completely, infringements on one's idealized self-image. In these events, embarrassment occurred because people behaved in a manner that was incompatible with their idiosyncratic, personal goals, not because they had done anything that was normatively incorrect. In one case, a 16-year-old was embarrassed when her mother found her necking with her boyfriend in a car in front of her house; she wrote, "I was embarrassed because I had my mother and entire family believing I was an angel and would never park with a boy. And here she caught me red-handed" (Cupach & Metts, 1990, pp. 344–345). Although her behavior was typical of teenagers, it was inconsistent with the way she wished to be judged, and so she was embarrassed by events that many of her peers would have considered routine.

Separately, the two classification schemes of Cupach and Metts (1990, 1992) and Miller (1992) were the most practical and useful on record. Together, they offered the most efficient but comprehensive means of cataloguing embarrassments available. Both research teams appreciated the clever contributions of the other (I can vouch for myself; see also Cupach & Metts, 1994), and the two schemes were reasonably compatible. A free lunch is hard to come by, however, and there was one thing standing in the way of a simple integration of the two models; both teams had developed their schemes on reports from people who described their embarrassments from memory. In their procedure, Cupach and Metts simply asked their respondents to describe an occasion that had caused them significant embarrassment (Metts & Cupach, 1989). With those instructions, more vivid and dramatic abashments that would readily spring to mind were undoubtedly more likely to be recalled. For instance, we've seen that a college student asked about embarrassment described being caught "parking" at the age of 16, a memorable example but one several years old. In my procedure, I asked people to tell me about their most recent embarrassment, guiding their memory search to more current events; nevertheless, strong, sensational embarrassments still were probably more likely to come to mind than more recent, mundane examples (see Thomas & Diener, 1990).

Our methods might have missed mild, rare embarrassments. To be more confident of detecting infrequent but meaningful predicaments, a more sensitive technique was desirable. Toward that end, Cathy Stonehouse and I decided to collect more data with which to integrate the two classification schemes. We hoped to obtain more reliable estimates of the relative frequencies with which these events occurred, and also suspected that one or two previously undetected categories of embarrassment might emerge. We were right.

We asked both college students and fifth-graders to keep track of their embarrassments over time with "embarrassment diaries" (Stonehouse & Miller, 1994). Once a week for 4 weeks (the fifth-graders) or 8 straight weeks (the college students), the students reported how often they had been embarrassed during the past week and provided details on their most recent embarrassment, if any. Embarrassment occurred frequently in these groups, with 94% of them, on average, being embarrassed by something each week; the typical respondent encountered 1.5 embarrassing experiences every 7 days. Overall, we examined 753 different accounts of embarrassment, and although various biases in reporting were still possible, I think we obtained the most comprehensive array of embarrassing circumstances ever. With them, we produced a new catalogue of embarrassments that integrated and improved upon past efforts (see Table 4.1).[1]

## HOW DO WE EMBARRASS?
## LET US COUNT THE WAYS

### Individual Behavior

Most of the embarrassments we experience result from real or imagined flaws in our own behavior. The most common broad source of embarrassment by far is "individual behavior," in which the embarrassed person's own conduct is the cause of dismay. In most such cases, the person's behavior has violated shared standards of deportment, civility, control, or grace, so that there is an obvious shortcoming in the person's actions. We called such events *normative public deficiencies* to emphasize that the person is guilty of some lapse that would be apparent to most observers.

*Normative Public Deficiencies*

The simplest and most common such deficiencies are *physical pratfalls/inept performances* in which people are unduly clumsy or incompetent. One of our respondents had trouble simply staying in his seat:

"I was sitting in my biology class listening to my professor's lecture. I leaned back in my seat and almost fell out. Unfortunately, everybody else in the classroom saw what happened, including the professor."

Another student ripped the top of a pool table with an errant pool cue, several people misplayed fly balls or tripped rounding third, and (in one of my personal favorites) a woman caught her "hair on fire by leaning over a bunsen burner during lab" (Miller, 1992, p. 193).

A remarkable variety of trips, slips, and spills fit this category, but for sheer salience and duration it's hard to beat this account from a correspondent to the teen magazine YM ("Say Anything," 1991/1992, p. 12)[2]:

TABLE 4.1. Categories of Embarrassment

|  | Frequency of occurrence |
|---|---|
| **Individual behavior** | |
| I.   Normative public deficiencies | |
|      A. Physical pratfalls/inept performances | 17% |
|      B. Cognitive errors | 15% |
|      C. Loss of control over: | |
|           1. One's body | 5% |
|           2. One's emotions | 2% |
|           3. One's possessions | 9% |
|      D. Failures of privacy regulation | 3% |
|      E. Abashed harmdoing | 5% |
| II.  Departures from personal goals | 2% |
| III. Conspicuousness | 2% |
| IV.  Undue sensitivity | 4% |
| **Interactive behavior** | |
| V.   Awkward interaction | |
|      A. Loss of script | 4% |
|      B. Guilty knowledge | 4% |
| VI.  Partner sensitivity | 1% |
| **Audience provocation** | |
| VII. Real personal transgression present | |
|      A. Others intend to embarrass | 1% |
|      B. Others do not intend to embarrass | |
|           1. Criticism/correction | 1% |
|           2. Inadvertent disclosures | 0.4% |
|           3. Miscellaneous action | 0.3% |
| VIII. No personal transgression | |
|      A. Others intend to embarrass | 6% |
|      B. Others do not intend to embarrass | |
|           1. Criticism/correction | 1% |
|           2. Excessive attention/overpraise | 1% |
|           3. Others' mistakes/loss of control | 3% |
|           4. Miscellaneous action | 0.3% |
| **Bystander behavior** | |
| IX.  "Team" transgressions | 10% |
| X.   Empathic embarrassment | 3% |

"My freshman year of high school I went to a big party where there were lots of juniors and seniors. Everyone was really excited because a popular band was going to perform. When the band started to play, the loud music startled me and I spilled my drink all over my shirt. I ran toward the bathroom, but I tripped over the band's electric cord and fell. They were cut off in mid-song, and there was complete silence until I was able to untangle myself and plug the cord back in."

Altogether, various physical mistakes of this sort were the single most common category of embarrassment, representing a full sixth (17%) of the embarrassments encountered by the young adults in our sample.

A second class of public deficiency involved various *cognitive errors*. Waiters who served the wrong food to patrons, lovers who called their current partners by their old partners' names, and students who were caught daydreaming by an instructor's question were guilty of cognitive errors. We did not formally distinguish among different kinds of these mistakes, but they generally seemed to be of four types. The first was a *mistake in judgment*. In one example of this, the genteel advice columnist Ann Landers was once served what she believed to be an "unusual lacy coconut dessert" (Morley, 1983, p. 72) at a formal dinner party. With great difficulty, she cut out a piece and was about to eat it when an astonished companion pointed out that it was a doily. In another example, one of our college respondents reported working hard, trying different keys with growing consternation, to drive away someone else's car. He finally realized his error and had to ask his date to move with him to *his* car, parked nearby. Finally, one person who probably would have been embarrassed, given the chance, was Union General John Sedgewick at the Battle of Spotsylvania Court House during the U.S. Civil War who said, surveying the enemy lines, "They couldn't hit an elephant at this dist—" Those were his last words (Petras & Petras, 1993, p. 146).

Other cognitive errors involved *forgetfulness*. On occasion, people failed to remember the most elementary facts, much like this college woman:

"I was giving my future mother-in-law some addresses for my bridal shower. I couldn't remember the address of one of my bridesmaids, so I told her I would call her back and tell her later. It wasn't until 3 days later when I realized that I did know her address, because I presently live with her. When I called and told her what the address was and how I found it, she just started laughing."

Other people were often the targets of poor memories as respondents fumbled or forgot others' names or even their entire identities. Author

Rona Jaffe was embarrassed when she told a date a story about a previous evening with a fellow who had been a dreadful bore, and then realized she was describing an earlier evening with the same date (Morley, 1983)!

Errors also resulted from *lack of attention* and *temporary stupidity.* Gene Roddenberry, the creator of the "Star Trek" television series, was addressing a learned audience in Huntsville, Alabama (where there are real rocket scientists), when he confused nuclear fission and fusion, getting them backwards (Morley, 1983). He was abashed by his mistake, as was, no doubt, an accused thief acting as his own lawyer who asked a trial witness, "Did you get a good look at my face when I took your purse?" (Petras & Petras, 1993, p. 105). The thief's abashment was complemented by conviction and a 10-year sentence.

Students were often embarrassed by their clumsy answers to classroom questions, and various malapropisms and verbal mistakes also fit this category. In other examples, consider a broadcaster for the San Diego Padres who introduced himself one night, "Hi, folks, I'm Jerry Gross. No, I'm not, I'm Jerry Coleman" (Petras & Petras, 1993, p. 173). When he was still Vice-President of the United States, George Bush noted, "For $7\frac{1}{2}$ years I've worked alongside President Reagan. We've had triumphs. Made some mistakes. We've had some sex . . . Uh . . . setbacks" (Petras & Petras, 1993, p. 71). Errors like these were immediately noticed, but on occasion people didn't seem to have been paying close attention to their own behavior; after an earthquake in February 1990, a Los Angeles disc jockey announced, "The telephone company is urging people to *please* not use the telephone unless it's absolutely necessary in order to keep the lines open for emergency personnel. We'll be right back after this break to give away a pair of Phil Collins concert tickets to caller number 95" (Petras & Petras, 1993, p. 194). Problems like these involving stupidity, forgetfulness, bad judgment, or lack of attention occurred frequently among our college students, accounting for one out of every seven (15%) of their embarrassing experiences.

A third broad class of normative public deficiency involved lapses of appropriate management or control over one's person or possessions. We termed these transgressions "loss of control," and because these predicaments could be of very different types, we distinguished between three distinct kinds of control problems. The first was *loss of control over one's body,* and included episodes of inadvertent flatulence, belching, hiccupping, and (because we surveyed a college population) many instances of intoxication. Here's a vivid but apt example:

> "On Wednesday, after our test, my friends and I wanted to celebrate. We went to [a local club] for Long Island Ice Teas. After we'd been there a couple of hours, I was feeling queasy, so my friends called

my boyfriend to come take me home. As he was walking me out to his car, I threw up all over his shirt."

You may be thinking that it shows bad judgment to poison oneself this way, and this woman's seemingly deliberate intoxication *was* ill-conceived. Nevertheless, her embarrassment was classified as a loss of control instead of a cognitive error due to a conceptual decision we made about our categorization strategy. When we were faced with predicaments that could be variously construed to fit more than one category, we opted to classify them according to the actual events that were apparent to the audience before whom embarrassment occurred. We considered the person's behavior from the *audience's perspective* and targeted the specific threat to the person's social identity in that situation. Procedurally, that meant we sometimes ignored the personal, private stream of thought respondents relayed to us in their accounts.

For instance, here is another loss of body control: "I was at a wedding and at the quietest moment my stomach growled *very loud*. I held my stomach hoping it would stop it. I knew I should have eaten." Privately, this respondent may blame herself for the bad decision of skipping lunch, but the only thing known to those sitting around her was that her stomach was out of control. We tried to characterize the *specific proximal public predicaments* our respondents faced, and thus coded the growling stomach as "loss of control" regardless of the prior behavior that may have led up to it.

As a final example of this point, one could argue that a person who (1) makes a bad decision to (try to) sneak an intestinal emission past unwitting companions, and who (2) is subsequently embarrassed when said emission is more noisome than anticipated, has committed a (private) cognitive error. Nevertheless, the public transgression, the event known to observers and the source of social disapproval, is a loss of control, and that would be the category applied. This strategy also had the desirable consequence of allowing us to ignore the private *intentions* people sometimes reported—which were, after all, known only to them—in favor of describing their overt *behavior*, which was obvious to everyone. Our categories were more reliable and our scheme had more utility as a result.

With this strategy in place, loss of control over one's body comprised 5% of the embarrassments we obtained. One more familiar example of such loss of control is noteworthy—dozing off at the wrong time or in the wrong place. In one exotic example, a college student who fell asleep in class awoke to find *an entirely different class* going on around him. Startled, he gathered his things and dashed out, with no one in the room seeming to pay him any attention; once the door shut behind him, though, he heard uproarious laughter from within.

A second, rarer, control problem was *loss of control over one's emotions*. About 2% of embarrassments fit this category, which always entailed stronger emotions than people felt were appropriate. A common example was excessive temper:

> "My little girl has recently learned to ride her bicycle without training wheels. She has not developed good judgment about safety rules so I have to watch her when she rides on the street. Monday, she was riding her bicycle and a car was backing out of a driveway as she was approaching on her bike. I yelled at her to stop but she just smiled and kept on riding. The car stopped but I was so frightened I kept screaming at her to stop. When I ran to stop her, I lost control and talked to her badly in front of a neighbor who was standing nearby. He just shook his head as if to say, 'Lady, cool it with the kid.' I was very embarrassed that I mishandled the situation, and she learned nothing from me but fear and ridicule and my neighbor witnessed it."

People were also embarrassed by excessive fear:

> "I was at the ROTC Rappel Tower getting ready to go off the skid for the first time. (The skid is a 6-inch-diameter pipe 50 feet in the air—you stand on it and fall off backwards then slide to the ground on a rope.) I was scared to death—my roommate was below me watching and my boyfriend and a classmate were on top of the tower trying to get me to go. I got so scared, I started shaking and crying. I'm not the type that likes to cry—*especially* in front of others."

Because bullying and cowardice are both undesirable, one can understand the embarrassment that resulted in these examples from engaging in such behavior. Interestingly, however, even acceptable behavior reflecting sensitivity and sympathy could be embarrassing if it was incompatible with one's desired social identity. Male college students were occasionally embarrassed by crying at sad movies. Such tenderness is good for people (see Leary & Miller, 1986) but the belief that "big boys don't cry" is widely held, so men could be embarrassed by appropriate behavior that they nevertheless considered normatively incorrect.

A last difficulty with control entailed *loss of control over one's possessions*. Failure to manage one's clothes fits this category, including the familiar example of an open zipper:

> "Friday I was embarrassed upon entering my 8:00 A.M. class. I slept till about 7:50 and ran to class and as soon as I walked in some male

friends began to laugh and poke at me rather seriously. They then told me my zipper was down. If I wouldn't have been late and there weren't many people there, it wouldn't have been that bad, but I was the last one to walk in and all the girls saw me. I reacted by walking out of class, zipping my zipper up and then returning to class; presented with a loud round of applause by both students and my professor. The embarrassment level I experienced was unexplainable."

A variety of split or ripped pants are possible and rough surf often gobbles up bikini tops, but one of the most intriguing clothing examples I've ever seen befell this teenager ("Nightmare," 1992, p. 14):

"At an amusement park, my boyfriend and I got on a ride that spins while the floor drops out, making you stick to the walls. I was wearing a bikini top, and it flew off when the floor fell down! Since my hands were stuck to the wall, I couldn't grab my bikini or cover my chest. I was spinning around topless, and everyone on the ride and in line could see me! The carnival operator had to stop the ride for me to retrieve my top."

Pets and cars were the other possessions that frequently went out of control. Actor William Shatner was embarrassed at a party when his Doberman puppy jumped from his arms into a pool and then, with muddy feet, put his paws on the beautiful white gown of Gloria Vanderbilt (Morley, 1983). Our student respondents were often embarrassed by their cars stalling in the middle of busy intersections. Overall, 1 of every 11 embarrassments (9%) fit this control category, so that altogether, the three types of loss of control—over one's person, emotions, and possessions—accounted for almost as many embarrassments (16%) as the physical pratfall category.

Two final types of normative public deficiency were possible. *Failures of privacy regulation* occurred whenever people insufficiently protected private thoughts or actions from public view. This often involved unintended nudity, as in this example ("Say Anything," 1993, p. 14):

"Nobody was home, so after taking a shower I walked out of the bathroom, totally naked, singing 'Tomorrow' at the top of my lungs. I came face to face with the real estate agent who was showing our house and two of his clients! I wanted to die!"

More than simple nudity was involved, however, because this category was appropriate whenever an acceptable private activity caused embarrassment by becoming public. Consider this account:

"This weekend I was coming home from a date around 1:30 A.M. and I stopped at a stoplight and a good song came on the radio and I started singing with it. After a while I looked over to my left and there were two girls in another car watching me, so I stopped singing and took off when the light turned green."

Failures of privacy regulation, which accounted for 3% of all embarrassments, occurred somewhat less often than the last kind of normative deficiency, *abashed harmdoing*. One out of 20 predicaments (5%) occurred when people were embarrassed by inconveniencing, insulting, embarrassing, or harming others. Writer Michael Bentine (quoted in Morley, 1983, p. 25) says this happened to him at a theatrical audition when he was listening to a woman singing onstage:

"Her voice was so awful that I turned to the man sitting beside me and remarked upon it. He replied very frostily, 'That is my wife.' Pink with confusion, I hastily stammered, 'I didn't mean her voice was awful, only the song she was singing.' To which he replied, 'I wrote it.' I slunk away."

Some unintended "harmdoing" was rather mundane (see Bennett & Dewberry, 1989); one student reported, "I went to a professor's office and knocked on the door. When he came to the door, I saw he had someone in the office. I was embarrassed for interrupting him." Other examples were more dramatic, including my own drenching of a new acquaintance with a soft drink (see Chapter 1) and this account of anonymous spittle from above:

"Yesterday I was on the fourth floor of the GPC building in the stairwell. I wanted to see how high up one could get so I went to the fifth floor and looked over the rail. It was a long way down. It seemed like a good time and place to experiment so while no one was around I gathered some saliva in my mouth and spit over the rail. Just as it left my mouth an old prof walked in a door on the first floor. All I remember is the splat of my spit and a slam of a door. I don't think I'll ever use the stairs again."

*Departures from Personal Goals*

In all of the categories I've covered thus far, people committed obvious public transgressions. By definition, their behavior breached normative standards of conduct and so was deficient in some way that was apparent to ordinary observers. However, more subtle individual misbehavior also occurred. At the suggestion of Cupach and Metts (1992), we looked for

and found several instances in which people were personally disap-
pointed by behavior that was not normatively incorrect. In such cases,
people acted in ways that were inconsistent with their idiosyncratic goals
but did not necessarily seem untoward to anyone else. No normative
public deficiency existed, but *personal* public deficiencies did.

Among our college respondents, disappointingly low test grades
often caused this type of chagrin:

> "After taking the test in our class, I was out checking my answers,
> and after checking the first half of the test I had already missed
> several. I myself felt ashamed so I didn't even check the second half.
> I was stunned."

Glaring academic failures would have fit the cognitive errors category,
but average performances that violated one's own standards were inconsistent with personal ideals.

Other departures from personal goals involved living rooms that
weren't clean enough, physiques that weren't slim enough, and drink-
ing that wasn't infrequent enough. Actor Walter Matthau (quoted in
Morley, 1983, p. 78) was even guilty of manners that he thought
weren't polished enough; when he met Eleanor Roosevelt, he was
nervous and:

> "I said the first words that came to mind—'Pleased to meet you.'
> That, sir, is the biggest gaffe I ever made. I was pleased to meet her,
> but to make such a casual remark was very embarrassing."

You can see that this category required us to judge whether a given
behavior was *normatively* incorrect or merely personally undesirable.
This category was used when a person engaged in ordinary behavior
much like that of others, but was embarrassed by it nonetheless. Mr.
Matthau might have wished to say, "My dear woman, to be in your
presence is inexpressibly delightful," but we thought that it was typical
for someone to say, "Pleased to meet you," and thus did not judge a
normative transgression to have occurred. Using this decision rule, such
departures from personal goals comprised 2% of the embarrassments we
obtained.

## Conspicuousness

Embarrassment usually entails a sense of exposure, and public misbehavior often catches others' attention. On occasion, however, people became the salient objects of the attention of others when they had not

misbehaved at all. When innocuous behavior nevertheless caused someone to stand out from the crowd, *conspicuousness* occurred.

Even when they had done nothing wrong, people didn't like to be obvious:

> "Tuesday was our last day of lab. We were to show up for a quiz, and then if we wished, we could stay for a review. Well, after we took our quiz and received our grades, *everyone* left the lab session, that is, everyone *except* me. I felt a little leery just sitting there waiting for the lab review to begin. I felt uncomfortable sitting there, so I began asking the lab instructor questions. At first, she was also uncomfortable, but after a couple of questions she warmed up and truly helped me review for my lab practical. Overall, *now* I am glad I stayed."

If people attracted attention through normatively deficient behavior, or had attention thrust upon them by the actions of others (e.g., the waiters' surprise rendition of "Happy Birthday to You" at a restaurant), other categories were appropriate. Simple conspicuousness in the absence of one's own or others' transgressions occurred 2% of the time.

### Undue Sensitivity

The last category of embarrassment resulting from individual behavior was one detected for the first time using our diary methodology (Stonehouse & Miller, 1994). People sometimes overreacted to ordinary events, becoming embarrassed in situations that, by normative standards, should not have been embarrassing. Such emotion seemed excessive and seemed to result from *undue sensitivity* to situations of only mild awkwardness:

> "My fiancée and me went to buy groceries. As we were walking the aisles, she reminded me that she was out of her monthly feminine items and proceeded to that section. Once she realized I was embarrassed, she started laughing and placed the box on top. Needless to say I quickly buried it in the basket of groceries."

One out of every 25 embarrassments (4%) fit this category. No normative deficiency could be said to occur in these cases, but people were still abashed on occasion by trivial failings:

> "Last Saturday at a bass tournament I fished all day in the rain and wind and didn't catch anything at all. Then, at 2:00 at the weigh-in, even though no one else had any fish to weigh in, while I was

standing there with no fish I felt a little bit embarrassed and awkward, even though only 12 people out of 365 people caught fish."

## Summary

Altogether, nearly two-thirds (64%) of the embarrassments encountered by the young adults in our sample resulted from individual behavior, and more than half (56%) followed some sort of normative public deficiency. Most of the time people had good reason to be embarrassed after their public pratfalls, mental mistakes, and losses of control; these were obvious lapses of normal decorum that were apparent to average audiences. Nevertheless, one of every 12 embarrassments (8%) resulted from individual action that was not obviously incorrect and that was not likely to engender social disapproval; in such cases, people were embarrassed by sheer conspicuousness or idiosyncratic failings, or simply seemed to overreact to routine events. There's a telling point here. Most embarrassments result from glaring public errors, but embarrassment is both more widespread and more subtle than that; it can emerge from various situations in which people behave tolerably well. No noticeable personal failing need arise for embarrassment to occur. Moreover, this becomes even clearer as we move from individual behavior to transactions in which others are more closely involved.

### Interactive Behavior

As we noted earlier, the appropriate focus for understanding some embarrassments is neither the individual conduct of the person who becomes embarrassed nor the actions of any observers; instead, some predicaments emerge from the *combined* behavior of two or more people, all of them individually blameless, in an ongoing interaction. In prototypical instances, an interaction becomes awkward or uncomfortable because of the particular people with whom one is conversing, but no normative misbehavior (on anyone's part) occurs. These are cases of *awkward interaction*, and they can be of two types.

## Awkward Interaction

The first type of interactive predicament is a *loss of script*. This occurred when people found themselves flustered and unsure of how to proceed as a result of the nature of, or some event within, an ongoing interaction. Even in the absence of some mistake, people sometimes lost their confidence and poise when they were faced with a maladroit situation. Some interactions started poorly:

> "I was riding in the car with a person whom I was not acquainted with and he had a speech impairment. I could not understand anything that this person was saying and did not know how to converse."

Other interactions took unanticipated, awkward turns:

> "On Monday night I received a phone call from my mother telling me that a friend from high school had committed suicide. This person was best friends for years with my old high school flame. Out of concern I called my old boyfriend to see if he was all right. We haven't spoken for a while and he is married with two children. I only called to make sure he was holding up well and offer my sympathy. During the conversation somehow it got off track and a lot of old feelings and memories were stirred up by him. Like he told me about the trouble in his marriage and what great eyes I had. I felt awkward and embarrassed due to the fact the reason I called was because of this tragedy. Maybe he was looking for a diversion. Me, I looked for a way out of the conversation."

Finally, the context of an interaction could suddenly change, with ill effect:

> "I was at [a local club] with some girlfriends and I was kinda flirting with a guy I've had in several classes. He had bought me a couple of beers and the next thing I know, I look up and here comes my boyfriend! I quickly told the guy that a guy I had been going out with (I didn't tell him we had been dating for 2 years) had just walked in. Everything turned out okay, but initially I wanted to hide."

Of the embarrassments reported to us, 4% were awkward interactions like these. Another 4% resulted from a second kind of interactive predicament, in which participants' *guilty knowledge* of past events adversely affected their current interactions. Whenever a person's private knowledge of a past incident made a present situation awkward or uncomfortable, this category pertained. Here's an example:

> "While in Dallas this past weekend, a friend and I ran into an old friend who recognized my friend (but at first not me). She introduced him to me. I remembered his name but could not place where I knew him from. My friend said, 'You know each other; remember,

y'all slept on my couch together once.' Then it dawned on me. He was a former lover. That night on the couch was more than just sleeping. Both of us had been extremely drunk and neither of us had remembered. When I figured out who it was, I started blushing hard. My face felt *so* red. I immediately hated myself for being in this situation. The guy kept putting his arm on, or around, me, smiling, and saying, 'Wow, that was crazy, huh?' I just smiled and tried to be polite and find a way to get away. Finally, he left."

In another case, a student assistant who had been roundly but correctly criticized by a supervisor felt awkward and uneasy in subsequent conversations with that supervisor.

Embarrassments involving guilty knowledge differed from those caused by a loss of script in that guilty knowledge always stemmed from past events whereas a loss of script issued from the current interaction itself. The difference is clear in one final, compelling example in which a case of loss of script became guilty knowledge a day later. A fellow wrote Ann Landers that he was packing for a first overnight trip with a new romantic partner and thought that he should be prepared; "I stopped by a drugstore to buy some condoms. I had never bought condoms before, so I was a little ill at ease. I tried to make small talk with the pharmacist and foolishly blurted out that I might 'get lucky' over the weekend" (Landers, 1994, p. 7G). His clumsy, scriptless interaction with the pharmacist was one thing, but you can imagine his guilty, embarrassed surprise the next morning when he went to pick up his date, rang her doorbell, and the pharmacist opened the door! His date was the pharmacist's daughter.

### Partner Sensitivity

Another rare category of embarrassment reported for the first time in our diary sample involved events that were ordinarily acceptable but that became embarrassing due to a unique audience's disapproval of such activity. The category assumed that no normative deficiency was demonstrated and that the audience's critical judgment was relatively unusual in finding fault where others would not. In such situations, then, no predicament would have occurred had different people been present, but the embarrassed person was correctly concerned about his or her image before the present audience. Thus it was the audience's standards that were unusual, not anyone's behavior, and audience, or *partner*, *sensitivity* was said to be the source of chagrin.

Such episodes usually occurred because someone was especially straitlaced or touchy. In one example, a middle-aged female student was chatting with a church friend when a much younger male student, who had been her neighbor for years, walked up, put his arm around her waist, and said, "Hey, darlin'." The woman had a history of such playfulness with the young man and was contentedly married, but the astonished, distressed look on the church friend's face caused her immediate embarrassment. Cases like these did not occur often and accounted for only 1% of all embarrassments, but they served to demonstrate once again that some embarrassments are not our fault.

## Audience Provocation

In fact, one out of every seven embarrassments our respondents encountered was thrust upon them by the actions of others. *Audience provocation* seemed an appropriate label for these situations, because in every case other people somehow singled out the embarrassed person for unwanted attention. In some cases, audiences intentionally sought to embarrass their victims, but more often, some other result was intended. Moreover, in most instances of audience provocation, the victim had committed no actual transgression that made embarrassment appropriate; in such cases, any embarrassment was truly the result of others' intervention.

### Personal Transgression Present

We distinguished between those cases in which the embarrassed person had misbehaved in some fashion and those in which no meaningful transgression was present. On occasion, *with intent*, people made a current audience aware of some past or present shortcoming of a person, publicizing or exaggerating some real transgression. These were either cases of playful teasing or overt hostility, but they occurred infrequently, accounting for only 1% of all embarrassments. More often (though still rarely overall), audience provocateurs publicized past predicaments *without* necessarily *intending to embarrass* their victims. One way this could occur was through *criticism* or *correction* offered by others. For instance, student workers were routinely embarrassed by even mild criticism if a supervisor delivered it when other coworkers were present. Audience members and interactive partners could also cause embarrassment without meaning to through *inadvertent disclosures*. Even well-meaning friends could unintentionally cause chagrin; as one student was carrying a full tray of food and drink at a pizza buffet, she

> "stumbled over a step. I did not fall, but one of my roommates stood up and shouted across the restaurant, 'Are you okay?' I was embarrassed because all the other people in the restaurant looked up to

see what was happening. I did appreciate my roommate's concern for my safety, but I wish she would not have shouted it out so loudly."

Partners also failed to keep secrets, letting embarrassing information slip out at inopportune times. We did not find that such slips were frequent, but they are apparently memorable; when Sandra Petronio and her colleagues at Arizona State University asked students to describe an incident in which a romantic partner had embarrassed them, a failure to keep a relational secret was mentioned by more than a third of the group (Petronio, Olson, & Dollar, 1989).

A small variety of *miscellaneous actions* by others could also exacerbate predicaments, and, altogether, unintentional audience provocation when real transgressions existed accounted for 2% of the embarrassments encountered by young adults.

*No Personal Transgression*

The most common provocation from an audience was teasing *with the intent to embarrass* when the victim had not actually done anything wrong. Often, this took the form of outright mocking, heckling, or razzing as in this example: "At my job, I have to wear a stupid straw cowboy hat. My boyfriend came in with his friend—they both sat, stared, and laughed." On other occasions, however, people were ensnared in deliberate, elaborate practical jokes (Miller, 1992, p. 194):

> "It was my senior year in high school. During a pep rally they wanted me to participate in a banana eating contest. All the contestants were blindfolded and given a banana in the middle of the gym (with everyone watching). But little did I know that after I was blindfolded that I would be the only one to participate. Eating a banana as fast as I could, blindfolded with the whole school cheering me on."

These were examples of what William Sharkey calls "intentional embarrassment," in which someone was deliberately singled out for embarrassing treatment. In his work at the University of Hawaii, Sharkey (1991) found that most adults (75%) had tried to embarrass somebody else at least once in the last 6 months, so events like these were well known. Moreover, in a survey of 1,136 people who were asked to describe a past attempt to embarrass someone, Sharkey (1992) was able to delineate six different tactics of intentional embarrassment. They included (1) the teasing and practical jokes noted above, and other manufactured predicaments such as (2) physical pratfalls, (3) violations of privacy, and (4) conspicuousness, along with excessive (5) criticism and deliberate (6) "team" transgressions (a category we consider below). We looked for all of these in our sample, curious about their relative frequency, but found that only teasing occurred with any regularity. Our sample reported 28 instances of teasing but only 6 examples of other tactics. Two pratfalls were created (e.g., a woman was thrown into a pool by her boyfriend) and two privacy violations occurred (one fellow was locked out of his house in his underwear, another had a bathing suit yanked down to his ankles). However, the remaining two examples seemed to fit a category of intentional embarrassment *not* discussed by Sharkey, "malicious intent"; in one case, a prison guard was embarrassed by vile trash talk from an inmate, and in the other, a woman was embarrassed by an anonymous rumor started by a coworker.

Overall, these events represented 6% of the embarrassments we analyzed. Intentional embarrassments are apparently familiar events, but they account for only a small fraction of the embarrassments people encounter.

A final group of audience provocations occurred when there was no personal transgression and the provocateurs apparently had *no intent to embarrass* their victims. Following the lead of Cupach and Metts (1992), we distinguished three different ways this occurred. One was *undue criticism*, which came out of thin air in this report: "I was at the shopping center and picked up a box of condoms. I had my daughter with me and a woman said, 'Why start using them now, it didn't work the first time.' I was stunned." (Audiences may have wished to *injure* their targets with such actions, but typically did not seem to wish to embarrass them.) Of the embarrassments experienced by our sample, 1% fit this category.

Another possibility was *excessive attention* or *overpraise*. Laura Buss (1978) had shown that too much acclaim could make people uncomfortable in the laboratory, and sure enough, lavish compliments did occasionally embarrass people. One woman wrote:

> "I was in Galveston for spring break with my boyfriend, and my uncle started asking him when he was going to marry me. My uncle was saying what a good catch I am and how sweet and pretty, and athletic and smart and on and on. I guess it was a good kind of embarrassment, but I'm just sort of modest, so I did feel somewhat awkward."

Unwanted attention or recognition of other kinds also seemed to fit this category. A college man was embarrassed when a woman he did not know well asked him to make love to her, and a teenager was embarrassed when her younger brother hid a video camera in her bathroom, filmed her in the nude, and then started selling copies of the tape for $10 each

("Say Anything," 1992). Episodes involving excessive attention or overpraise did not occur often, accounting for only 1% of all embarrassments, but it is still intriguing that they occurred. They are very different from the obvious pratfalls and errors that are often thought to characterize embarrassing circumstances; not only is there no normative deficiency in cases of overpraise, there is no hint of possible social disapproval. If anything, the embarrassed person is getting too much *favorable* attention. Moreover, such events appear to be genuinely embarrassing; they appear rarely, but reliably, in self-reports of embarrassment (cf. Miller, 1992), and when asked to decide, most people agree with the statement, "I can be embarrassed when I am complimented or praised by others" (Parrott & Harré, 1991). When we explore the reasons *why* all these circumstances embarrass us in our analysis of the psychological sources of embarrassment in Chapter 7, we will have to consider the singular category of overpraise closely.

Other unintentional, undeserved embarrassments resulted from *mistakes* or *losses of control* from audience members. Unfortunate victims were sometimes on the receiving end of others' normative public deficiencies and were embarrassed by their inept behavior. One woman was goosed and twirled around by a man who said, "Whoops! You're not who I thought you were"; another had to ward off the blunt sexual invitations of an inebriated acquaintance—another woman's fiancé—at a night club; and yet a third was being introduced to an otherwise charming and attractive young professor/author when he accidentally dumped a large soft drink on her head at a busy campus eatery. Of the embarrassments reported to us, 3% were of this sort.

When a small collection of *miscellaneous actions* were included (e.g., one fellow stepped out of the shower to find that his roommate had unlocked the bathroom door to let his girlfriend in; there she was, sitting on the toilet), more than 5% of all embarrassments fit this whole group of unintended, undeserved embarrassments caused by others. Overall, as the audience provocations clearly show, quite a few episodes of embarrassment simply were not the victims' fault.

## Bystander Behavior

At least in the audience provocations, the embarrassed victims were the unambiguous targets of the behavior of the provocateurs. For instance, the fellow chosen as the butt of the joke in the high school banana eating contest was obviously singled out for special treatment. However, one last broad type of embarrassments afflicted people who were merely *bystanders* of others' embarrassing actions and who were not necessarily personally involved in the action at all. This class of embarrassing circumstances demonstrated that simply participating in social life, even when one's own behavior was flawless, could result in eventual embarrassment.

### "Team" Transgressions

Out of every 10 embarrassments, 1 occurred when people were with someone else who did something embarrassing. In *"team" transgressions* a person's associates misbehaved, and—although no personal deficiencies were demonstrated—the person was evidently concerned that third-party observers would judge the team members' actions to reflect negatively on him or her. Most parents who have spent much time in public with their children are probably familiar with this category of embarrassment; in one example:

> "I was in a large mall with my brother-in-law and my 5-year-old nephew when a rather well-endowed lady was walking our way. When she got about 3 feet from us my nephew said, as loud as he could, 'Look at those tits, Dad!' Extremely embarrassing."

On the other hand, parents occasionally embarrassed their children as well:

> "I was talking on the phone to a friend when my mother farted. He asked if it was me that made the noise because it was a loud echoing sound. So I had to tell him it was my mother stepping on a frog."

Family members were often the authors of team transgressions —in fact, humorist Dave Barry argues that "Your most important responsibility, as the parent of an adolescent, is to be a hideous embarrassment to your child" (1994, p. 15)—but, among our college sample, friends were actually the more common culprits. In one such case:

> "I went to my hometown this past weekend and my friend and I were driving around after we had been out partying. We were at a stop light and when the light turned green my friend gassed her truck and ran into the car in front of us. Although there was no damage done to either car I was embarrassed because the car she ran into was one of my friends in high school—who I haven't seen since graduation."

### Empathic Embarrassment

In team transgressions, one might feel guilty by association, at least in others' eyes. In contrast, in a final specific category of embarrassment, bystanders could be abashed even when *no* connection existed between themselves and another person's predicament. When people felt embarrassment for others whose actions did not reflect on them and with whom—in an audience's judgment—they were not associated, *empathic embarrassment* was said to occur. Just as Sattler (1965) suggested, and as I found in the lab (Miller, 1987), people could be greatly affected by watching the public abashments of others: "My professor made a fool of himself in front of the class, and I felt embarrassed and sorry for him because everyone laughed at him!"

Arguably, this was the most subtle form of embarrassment. Even when others were not aware of their own predicaments and were not distressed at all, bystanders could feel empathic embarrassment for them by imagining themselves in the same situation:

"I was walking behind a girl on campus who had on a skirt about knee-length and her slip was showing below the skirt by about 3 inches. As I walked behind her I could hear people laughing and saying, 'Someone please tell her!' I felt so badly for her but I didn't want to tell her because I knew that she'd be humiliated. So I felt embarrassment for her by thinking how upset I would be."

(Interestingly, had this respondent not felt empathic embarrassment she might have been able to coolly inform the girl about her predicament and end it right there; unfortunately, as we'll see in Chapter 9, embarrassment often keeps people from doing things it would be good for them to do.)

Obvious displays of embarrassment from another person were clearly not necessary for witnesses' empathic embarrassment to occur. In fact, I was intrigued to find an example of a person feeling chagrin from simply *imagining* someone else's public predicament[3]:

"Three days ago, a friend of mine told me what it was like for her boyfriend to receive a singing telegram on his birthday. It was during class here at the University, by the way. The singers dressed up as cartoon characters and sang with masks covering half their faces. I just laughed so hard. I was embarrassed for him and knew how awkward he must have felt. Other people did not think it was embarrassing at all."

Such episodes aptly illustrate the pervasiveness and possible subtlety of embarrassment in daily life. Three percent of the embarrassing events experienced by our sample involved empathic embarrassment, and overall, people were abashed as mere bystanders in about one out of every eight embarrassing circumstances.

## CONCLUSIONS

This has been a long, but I hope worthwhile, chapter. The categorization scheme described here is certainly not the only one available; a variety of simpler efforts exist (see Anderson & Kauffman, 1991; Kauffman & Anderson, 1992; Sharkey & Stafford, 1990). These alternatives are a bit too simple, however, because they fail to illustrate some of the dimensions of embarrassment that emerge from the Stonehouse and Miller (1994) categories. I submit that our catalogue of embarrassments is the most useful on record. Its mutually exclusive categories encompass all the routine embarrassments people encounter and explicate several uncommon predicaments, as well.

Obviously, embarrassment can result from myriad events, and their diversity sets the stage for answers to vital questions about this pervasive social emotion. As we've seen, we can be personally embarrassed by our own mistakes, by those of our associates, *and* by those we see made by strangers. A catalogue of embarrassments like this begs the question of what it is about these various circumstances that makes them so arousing. The numerous embarrassments I've described here will necessarily play key roles in the evaluation of competing theoretical explanations of why embarrassment occurs. That's coming in Chapter 7.

Furthermore, as you considered these diverse predicaments, you may have wondered whether you would have responded to them as their authors did. The answer, of course, is "Maybe." Real differences exist among people that make some of us more susceptible to embarrassment than others are. It's conceivable that not all of these circumstances are embarrassing for all of us all of the time, and we'll have to take a close look at the personality traits that make that so. That's coming in Chapter 6.

Another important issue comes first. How do we learn to be embarrassed by these various circumstances? Any parent knows that a 4-year-old can be completely unconcerned by a violation of privacy that would humiliate an older sibling. Over time, children ordinarily learn to fear embarrassing predicaments that previously had no influence on them at all. Why does this occur? Should you want this to happen to your children? As we'll see in our next chapter, the answer to this last question is "Yes."

# CHAPTER 5

# The Development
# of Embarrassment

⮵

Do you remember that period in early childhood when you could not be embarrassed? It's unlikely that you can. It was long ago, but you, like all of us, were once immune to embarrassment. There was a time when you really didn't care what others thought of you. In fact, there was a time when you really couldn't *comprehend* what others thought of you, much less master the subtleties of polite interaction by which you might be judged.

However, this period of invulnerability to embarrassment occurred before the age at which you began to form the earliest memories that you can now recall. Most people's memories date back to age 3 or so (Bjorklund, 1989), and we are probably capable of a rudimentary form of embarrassment by then, so we generally cannot remember having once been unembarrassable. Still, when we were very young children, nothing could embarrass us.

Some other emotions emerge within months of birth, but because it depends on complex cognitive abilities that take years to develop, embarrassment gradually unfolds over time. Further, unlike other emotions, embarrassment seems to depend on the experiences children encounter. It may take years to provide a child enough teaching and training for him or her to feel embarrassment the way adults do.

These facts put embarrassment into a unique class of emotions and deserve close consideration. However, the precise manner in which embarrassment emerges is still a matter of debate. As we will see, some observers place the appearance of embarrassment as early as 18 months of age, but others argue that children are 10 years old before they are likely to experience the mature embarrassment that is the focus of this book. One thing is clear; regardless of its timeline, emerging embarrassment is molded by three monumental developmental influences: self-consciousness, cognitive development, and socialization.

## THE EMERGENCE OF SELF-CONSCIOUSNESS

Emotion researchers generally believe that humans are born with the capacity to be startled and to experience pleasure and distress; thereafter, several basic emotions such as fear, anger, joy, and surprise quickly emerge within the first few months of life (Lazarus, 1991; Lewis, 1993). An infant has an emotional life that is responsive to its environment, and it slowly learns to control that environment as motor control improves. What an infant doesn't have is a self-concept. A baby doesn't know whether it is a boy or girl, cannot organize judgments or opinions about who or what it is, and, consequently, cannot even recognize itself in a mirror.

This latter assertion may surprise some parents, but it is true. Our human capacity for self-recognition, our ability to consider ourselves, to examine our images and know, "That is I, distinct and unique from others," is a defining element of consciousness, but we're not born with it. Using a variety of ingenious techniques, researchers have shown that human infants are usually 1½ to 2 years old before they realize that the images they see in a mirror are their own reflections (Lewis & Brooks-Gunn, 1979).

This work has been fascinating and warrants a bit of explanation. Because mirrors are entertaining and youngsters will often inspect them closely, a key issue is how to determine that self-recognition has occurred in toddlers whose language skills are nascent. Gordon Gallup, Jr. (1970) pioneered a procedure in which chimpanzees who had experience with mirrors were anesthetized and painted with a bright red, odorless dye along an eyebrow and on top of an ear. When they awoke, the animals were carefully observed to see how often they touched the paint marks without a mirror present. (They almost never did.) When the mirror was returned, however, and they saw the marks—in their reflections—for the first time, they promptly touched, rubbed, and scratched the spots, even sniffing their fingers to test the dye's smell. Each clearly recognized that the face in the mirror was its own.

Gallup concluded that the chimpanzees' use of their reflections demonstrated self-recognition, a special talent that was later found to be limited to the great apes and humankind (Gallup, 1977, 1979).

However, similar studies with human infants demonstrated that reliable self-recognition is completely absent in 1-year-olds; it gradually emerges over the second year of life so that most children (about 75% of them) recognize themselves by their second birthday (Gallup, 1979; Lewis & Brooks-Gunn, 1979).

This is a developmental milestone that seems to mark the point at which children can begin to form organized beliefs about themselves as unique people, separate and different from others; this is when their self-concepts begin to form (Stipek, Gralinski, & Kopp, 1990). Children also begin to differentiate the sexes and to identify themselves as boys or girls at about the same age; until then, they haven't known *what* they were, or cared (Thompson, 1975). Typical 2-year-olds are thus beginning to think about themselves in entirely new, increasingly sophisticated ways. They are *self-conscious* in the sense that they are now able to analyze and judge themselves, thinking of themselves as male or female, good or bad, happy or sad. It is at just this point, some observers argue, that openness to embarrassment begins.

## Youthful Signs of Embarrassment

The first empirical study of the development of embarrassment in children was conducted by Arnold Buss and his colleagues at the University of Texas in Austin (A. H. Buss, Iscoe, & Buss, 1979). They contacted hundreds of parents of preschool or elementary school children, and asked whether they had noticed any signs of embarrassment in their children within the last 6 months. If a child had mentioned embarrassment to the parent or if the parent had noticed any blushing, silly giggling, nervous laughter, or hands covering the mouth, embarrassment was presumed to have occurred. With these criteria, 26% of a 3- and 4-year-old age group, 59% of 5-year-olds, and 73% of 6-year-olds had recently been embarrassed, and Buss et al. concluded that "embarrassment begins for most children at 5 years of age" (p. 229).

An obvious drawback of these data, of course, is that they were based on parents' recollections of their children's behavior. The parents had to notice and then remember reactions that looked embarrassed to them in order for any embarrassment to be reported to the researchers. Michael Lewis and his colleagues at the Robert Wood Johnson Medical School in New Jersey felt that an experience of embarrassment could be identified more directly, even in children too young to tell you what they were feeling, through careful observation of a child's pattern of behavior.

Lewis, Sullivan, Stanger, and Weiss (1989) thus watched children 1 year, 1½ years, or 2 years of age for signs of embarrassment. In one phase of their study, each child was suddenly confronted with his or her reflection in a large mirror. If smiling, gaze aversion, and nervous hand movements all occurred, the toddler was assumed to be embarrassed. Now, this is a key assumption that should not be accepted without a moment's deliberation. These nonverbal behaviors *are* classic indications of embarrassment in adults (Edelmann & Hampson, 1981b; Keltner, 1995), particularly when they occur in the right sequence (Asendorpf, 1990). When adults exhibit such behavior, they'll also say they're embarrassed. However, similar expressions in Lewis et al.'s procedure may not necessarily have indicated that the children were experiencing embarrassed emotion. Their behavior may have been merely bashful or coy. Had they suddenly been confronted with another child, their behavior might have been similar.

Nevertheless, Lewis et al. (1989) asserted that some of the toddlers *were* embarrassed, both because they looked like they were and because these signs of embarrassment were accompanied by evidence of self-recognition. In another phase of the investigation, the children were given a mirror self-recognition test; their mothers pretended to wipe their faces but dabbed nonscented rouge on their noses instead, and then placed them in front of a mirror. Signs of embarrassment and self-recognition tended to co-occur. Both were rare in the younger children, and both became more frequent with age; moreover, only 20% of the children who looked embarrassed did not also exhibit clear signs of self-recognition. Thus, the behavior that was thought to signal embarrassment corresponded with the emergence of self-consciousness. This is a telling datum because embarrassment is widely considered to be a state that cannot occur unless one is self-conscious (Tangney & Fischer, 1995).

However, only eight 2-year-old children participated in Lewis et al.'s (1989) first study (with five of them looking embarrassed), so a second investigation employed a larger sample and examined the children's responses to a wider variety of situations. Forty-four toddlers, all of them about 22 months old, were observed in front of a mirror with and without rouge on their faces. They also were given lavish compliments by the experimenter in an attempt to embarrass them through overpraise, and were coaxed to dance by the experimenter, who shook a small tambourine. A quarter of the children looked embarrassed when they saw their mirror images, and a third of them looked embarrassed by the praise and the conspicuous dancing (Lewis et al., 1989).

Most of these children also participated in a follow-up study a year later when they were 35 months old (Lewis, Stanger, Sullivan, & Barone, 1991). At 22 months, only 60% had exhibited self-recognition in the mirror test, but all of them displayed it when they were almost 3. Once again, 25–35% of the children exhibited signs of embarrassment when they were shown their reflections or effusively complimented, proportions that were no different than they had been a year earlier. The experimenter's request for a dance was apparently more daunting, however, because more than half of the children (57%) now looked embarrassed when faced with the public performance.

On the one hand, this increase in the embarrassing potential of the dance request—a situation that would certainly be embarrassing to most adults (see Apsler, 1975; Miller, 1987)—supports Lewis's argument that the animated behavior of the children is indicative of real embarrassment. On the other hand, a sizable minority of the children did not react to the dance request with signs of embarrassment despite having obviously attained self-consciousness. Moreover, it is still hard to know what to make of the claim that coy behavior in front of a mirror demonstrates that some 2-year-olds are embarrassed by their reflections. A mirror image does not ordinarily embarrass adults.

## Two Forms of Embarrassment?

In further defense of his claims, Lewis (1993, 1995) suggested that the sheepishness that coincides with self-recognition in 2-year-olds *is* embarrassment, but of a sort that does not perfectly resemble adult chagrin. For Lewis, early embarrassment is an emotion of mere exposure and conspicuousness, not one of social evaluation. He reasons that simple conspicuousness is a known cause of adult embarrassment (which is true) and that the emergence of self-consciousness around age 2 makes feelings of conspicuousness possible in young children. At that point, events that make a child a salient focus of attention, even to him- or herself in a mirror, cause the shrinking chagrin of real embarrassment. Not until age 3, says Lewis, do children slowly develop the capacity to evaluate their behavior with regard to shared social standards of conduct. It is then that shame, guilt, and a *second form* of embarrassment, which includes components of failure or transgression, are seen for the first time. This later type of embarrassment, which Lewis (1995) refers to as "mild shame," involves negative evaluation that is not necessarily present in the embarrassment that springs from mere exposure.

The position that there may be two forms of early embarrassment is not at all outrageous. In fact, there is an interesting precedent in shyness, which also seems to come in two varieties (A. H. Buss, 1986). Some children have a temperament that makes them wary and anxious around people who are unfamiliar to them (Kagan, Snidman, & Arcus, 1992); their inhibited behavior with strangers is apparent in their first year of life, and is called *fearful shyness* (Cheek & Briggs, 1990). In a very real sense, such children—representing about one out of every seven newborns (Kagan & Reznick, 1986)—are born shy. Fearful shyness has a strong genetic component (Plomin & Daniels, 1986), and shy children seem to have a sympathetic nervous system that causes greater arousal in strange situations than that experienced by uninhibited children (Kagan et al., 1992). Later on, after the emergence of self-consciousness, some children develop an awkward dread of social interaction that is based on concern about what others will think of them. This is *self-conscious shyness* (A. H. Buss, 1986). It is presumed to begin around age 5 in some people and to become most prevalent in adolescence when social evaluative concerns reach their peak (Cheek, Carpentieri, Smith, Rierdan, & Koff, 1986).

Data support the existence of these two developmental paths for adult shyness (e.g., Bruch, Giordano, & Pearl, 1986), so it is not particularly daring to suggest that both an "embarrassment of exposure" and an "embarrassment of deficiency" exist as well. One remaining problem, however, is the question of how exposure and conspicuousness are aversive to a 2-year-old. What is it about one's reflection in a mirror that causes embarrassed chagrin?

One possibility is suggested by existentialists such as Jean Paul Sartre who felt that it must be painful for people to come to view themselves as others do. Consciously adopting the perspective of others interrupts one's normal experience, so that taking "myself-as-object" is "an uneasiness, a lived wrenching away from the ecstatic unity of the for-itself" (Sartre, 1956, p. 251). Perhaps, then, the emergence of self-consciousness (of which a toddler is always reminded by his or her reflection) causes discomfort as the youngster faces the portentous insight of his or her individuality and separateness. This is less silly than it sounds. There are real burdens to selfhood (Baumeister, 1986, 1991), and after 2 years of symbiotic unity with Mom and Dad, the siblings, and one's favorite stuffed animal, it must be a dramatic change to look in a mirror and have a first rudimentary grasp of the implications of the reflected image.[1]

Still, even if such existential pain exists, why is *embarrassment* the emotion that results? Beulah Amsterdam and Morton Levitt (1980) provided one answer by suggesting that the emergence of self-consciousness is accompanied by more than simple conspicuousness. During that period of their lives, both boys and girls engage in regular play with their genitals. One influence that helps create self-consciousness, according to Amsterdam and Levitt, is the contrast between the personal pleasure attached to such play and the external scolding that typically results when parents notice it: "Painful self-consciousness develops as children are either quietly restrained and distracted, or more directly chastised and punished for exhibiting their bodies (nakedness) and for looking, touching, and playing with their genitalia" (p. 77). No sooner do typical children become self-aware, then, than they are instructed that their normal, enjoyable behavior is wrong. A sense of deficiency *does* accompany early conspicuousness as "the pleasurable sense of being, in which one is merged not only with the mother, but also with the universe, is lost, as one becomes an object of one's own observation, and the gleam in the mother's eye is transformed into an accepting, bewildered, or troubled look" (Amsterdam & Levitt, 1980, p. 82).

From this perspective, the early "embarrassment of exposure" identified by Lewis (1993, 1995) would be little different than the embarrassments exhibited by older children who are faced with overt predicaments; embarrassment would not have two forms. Early or later, it could be said to result from acute (if vague) concern regarding how one will be treated by significant others. Instances of self-recognition could remind a 2-year-old of the global difficulty he or she faces in eliciting consistent approval from others, and over time such concern might become more clearly associated with specific violations of social norms. This would explain the patterns in Lewis et al.'s (1991) data in which a dance request from a stranger embarrassed more 3-year-olds than 2-year-olds, while a mirror image (which might not remind secure children of any parental disregard) continued to embarrass only a small minority of children.

This analysis is admittedly speculative but it has the advantage of positing the continuous development of a single form of embarrassment from its origins in self-consciousness to its later association with specific adult predicaments. By comparison, Lewis's (1995) position is more complex, postulating an early type of embarrassment that "is captured, in yet unexplained ways" (p. 31) by a different, evaluative embarrassment that emerges later.

However, there is no evidence that will allow us to decide conclusively which is the better model, and in fact both may be entirely incorrect. The similarities between adult embarrassment and the behavior of 2-year-olds at a mirror may not indicate that the toddlers are embarrassed at all. Instead, as we noted earlier, the smiling and gaze aversion of the children may be nothing more than coy bashfulness. Over time, however, when youngsters blunder into various transgressions, they may discover that sheepish expressions consistently result in better treatment from others than do possible alternatives such as placidity or defiance. They may learn that apparent sheepishness has utility that makes it a desirable reaction to social predicaments, which in turn would make it increasingly commonplace in older children who encounter such situations. In this sense, the meaning of the expressions would change over time, and they would reliably reflect real embarrassment only in older children who had had sufficient social seasoning.

This "change-of-meaning" hypothesis permits us to dodge the question of whether 2-year-olds really get embarrassed by either exposure or existential pain (because there would be no way to tell), but it assumes that social experience plays a huge role in shaping the nonverbal expression of embarrassment, and that may not be true. Embarrassment looks much the same from culture to culture (Edelmann, 1990b) and is more consistent than one would expect if such expressions resulted mostly from social experience. My point in mentioning the meaning hypothesis is simply to remind you that several possibilities do exist and uncertainties remain.

Still, there are points of agreement. It seems clear that there are no signs whatsoever of embarrassment in young children until they become self-conscious. Psychoanalytic theorists believe that the related emotion of shame can be present from the moment of birth (e.g., Kaufman, 1989; Nathanson, 1987), but they provide no data to support their supposition, and it unquestionably falls outside the mainstream of empirical emotion research. In any case, no form of embarrassment appears until self-recognition is obtained (Lewis et al., 1989). It is also certain that embarrassment continues to unfold over time, so that children's responses to an embarrassing situation may change as they age (Lewis et al., 1991). This fact denotes the importance of two additional influences on the development of embarrassment on which theorists agree (e.g., A. H. Buss, 1980; Lewis, 1993): socialization and cognitive development.


## SOCIALIZATION

If children don't know the rules of social conduct, they are unlikely to be embarrassed by breaking them. When she was 2 years old, a friend of mine left her house on a fine spring day and walked several blocks downtown completely naked. When her family caught up with her, she was unfazed by her conduct and thought nothing was wrong. Of course, her family taught her otherwise (and *now* this story embarrasses her).

Naturally, all children must be taught the predominant values, standards, and norms of their cultures. They need to learn the rules, and the processes through which this occurs are termed *socialization*. Importantly, although people often conceive of emotions as biologically based, inborn response potentials, there is widespread agreement that emotional expressions and experiences are also modifiable through teaching and training (Saarni, 1993). For instance, a culture is likely to have both specific "feeling rules" (Hochschild, 1979) that suggest what one ought to feel in a given situation, and specific "display rules" (Ekman, 1972) that prescribe what emotions one should reveal. Thus, we've learned that we're not supposed to be gleeful at a funeral even if the deceased was a hated rival; if we are secretly pleased, we should at least respect the display rule and try to *look* mournful even though we're not. As Michael Lewis and Carolyn Saarni (1985, p. 15) asserted, "the biology of human beings disposes us to emotional, as well as cognitive and social behavior, [but] the nature of that behavior, the situations that elicit it, the things we feel, and whether we feel or not are all dependent on an elaborate set of socialization rules." On the whole, then, theorists generally accept the notion that, although the *capacity* for emotional experiences may be inborn, "the social matrix determines *which emotions are likely to be experienced when and where, on what grounds and for what reasons, by what modes of expression, by whom*" (Kemper, 1993, pp. 41–42).

## Socializing Embarrassment

Embarrassment is undoubtedly like other emotions in this regard. Self-consciousness may provide the foundation for embarrassment, but children must gradually learn when embarrassed reactions are appropriate and exactly what expressions others consider acceptable. How does such "emotional education" (Buck, 1991) proceed? Socialization of emotions (or anything else) is thought to involve all types of learning, which Saarni (1993) groups into "direct" and "indirect" influences. *Direct methods* of socialization are aimed directly at the person being trained and include classical conditioning (or learning through association), operant conditioning (shaping behavior through rewards and punishments), and didactic teaching (e.g., "You should be ashamed of yourself"). According to Arnold Buss (1980), all of them are key components in the socialization of embarrassment.

Soon after his or her second birthday, Buss believes, a youngster finds that certain behavior is likely to engender laughter, teasing, and ridicule from others. These are painful punishments that signal some transgression; they also cause embarrassment that quickly becomes associated with the violation. The first behavior regulated in this way, according to Buss, is the self-control of bladder and bowels. Once they are toilet trained, children are at risk of merciless taunting and teasing for any lapse of self-control. As a result, they quickly learn to dread any such accidents, and begin to react to them with embarrassment when they do occur.

Similar training in modesty and manners follows shortly thereafter. Nakedness, once an ordinary event, becomes tightly constrained. One learns to pick one's nose in private. Indoctrination in social standards never stops, and ultimately, subtle issues of privacy are learned. Older children find that some thoughts and activities (e.g., masturbation) should be carefully protected lest ridicule and disdain result. (As a matter of fact, when I was in fourth grade, I certainly came to regret telling some male classmates of my crush on our attractive, young, single teacher; they told *her*, and I had never been so embarrassed. It's best, I learned, to keep some feelings to yourself.)

Buss asserts that socialization of this sort has important consequences. One is that people may justifiably come to fear excessive attention from others because it is more often associated with disapproval and pain than with approbation and admiration. As a result, simple conspicuousness can become embarrassing, even in the absence of some normative deficiency; during childhood,

> a tight link is forged between conspicuousness and embarrassment. When a child is singled out, he or she is usually made to feel embarrassment. After hundreds of repetitions, conspicuousness becomes so closely associated with embarrassment that close scrutiny by others can cause embarrassment. (A. H. Buss, 1980, p. 233)

This link between simple conspicuousness and embarrassment probably results in a lot of needless social anxiety, and I think it's unfortunate. Nevertheless, as we saw in Chapter 4, the link does exist and its power can be impressive. I gave a talk on embarrassment to an audience of gifted junior high school students a while back, and was met with both the intelligent questions and brash braggadocio one sometimes finds in such groups. One particularly outspoken (actually, loud-mouthed) male claimed to be unembarrassable, and though that seemed to be true, I called his bluff. I asked all the other 17 students to turn and gaze directly at him, silently, for 45 seconds. All they did was look. The fellow resolutely accepted this at first, but soon looked down, hunched his shoulders, shifted in his seat, and blushed a bright red. Frankly, I was as surprised as he was, but it was a tremendous demonstration (and he was much more polite thereafter).

Michael Lewis (1995) elicits similar reactions from college students. To demonstrate the power of conspicuousness, he first forewarns an audience that he will close his eyes and then point out someone at random. When he does so, that person is invariably embarrassed even though there is obviously nothing personal connected to his choice of victim. Let me remind you, though, that Lewis interprets such effects as evidence of an embarrassment based on simple exposure that emerges very early and then continues throughout our lives. A. H. Buss (1980) suggests instead that conspicuousness gradually becomes embarrassing as it is associated with ridicule over and over again.

Thus both classical conditioning and operant conditioning may be central components of the socialization of embarrassment. Emotional education involves other important processes as well, described by Saarni (1985, 1993) as *indirect methods* of socialization. These include imitation, identification, and social referencing, and are said to be indirect because the relevant events are not specifically targeted at the person whose behavior is being changed. "Social referencing" refers to the manner in which one's own emotions can be influenced by knowledge of the feelings others are experiencing; in particular, when children are faced with ambiguous or novel situations, their emotional reactions are likely to resemble those they observe in others. Remarkably, even very young children are influenced by this process of observational learning; Feinman and Lewis (1983) showed that the reactions of 8-month-old infants to a stranger tended to match their mothers' emotional reactions to him.

Both imitation and social referencing probably cause children to learn from *others'* embarrassments as well as their own. Youngsters need not break the rules themselves to find out what they are. When others become embarrassed after some transgression and, worse, are taunted by observers for their mistakes, their examples delineate the rules and the consequences of breaking them. Straightforward principles of modeling thus predict that children could come to dread embarrassing circumstances they have merely witnessed and not even participated in themselves. These and other processes of "emotional contagion" (Hatfield, Cacioppo, & Rapson, 1993) also provide an explanation for the emergence of empathic embarrassment. As Eleanor Maccoby and John Martin (1983) noted, "when children repeatedly experience situations in which their affective state is matched to, or shared with, that of another person, this provides the conditions for the acquisition of conditioned empathic emotional responses" (p. 81). Young children may watch the predicaments of others with either dispassion or glee. However, as they gain experience in similar situations and gradually refine their abilities both to understand others' points of view and to decode their expressions, they become increasingly susceptible to empathic embarrassment. It may take years, but the socialization of embarrassment is so thorough that many people ultimately become susceptible to a personal discomfort that follows *observed* accidents and mistakes but does not involve either personal exposure or deficiency.

A final outcome of socialization is that children slowly come to accept and internalize any social rules that have been consistently enforced. Saarni (1985) explained this process of "identification." At first, because it is profitable to do so, children try to accommodate the stated expectations of their parents and other powerful authorities regarding what feelings are right and what feelings are wrong in various situations. On their own, they might be delighted if, by pulling a package of toilet paper from a grocery store display, they cause the whole stack to tumble to the floor; if an attentive parent is nearby, however, they quickly learn that a look of chagrin will provide better results than a delighted giggle. On the whole, children may try to model their emotions after those of older authorities because they are rewarded for doing so. Over time, though, these imitative behaviors take root and children come to believe that the authorities' expectations are appropriate; they then accept them as their own. Thereafter, a child's new personal standards can generalize to novel but similar situations in which no authority figure is present. In such a fashion, children gradually become embarrassed by misbehavior that might once have pleased them, and adhere to others' standards of conduct even when those others are absent.

## The Net Results

Altogether, it's easy to argue that these are desirable processes, despite the discomfort that embarrassment brings. By training children to be embarrassed by their mistakes, we reinforce appropriate standards of conduct that we generally *want* people to observe. Parents are probably pleased when their children finally internalize the rules and become more trustworthy; as Semin and Papadopoulou (1990, p. 110) noted, "child-rearing without the acquisition of such emotions would be a very difficult business" because youngsters would require constant supervision. Indeed, Gibbons (1990) stressed that the fear of embarrassment that results from normal socialization is very useful to society because it helps keep people from engaging in undesirable behavior; without embarrassment, he warned, "there would be social anarchy, and social discourse, as it exists, would be virtually impossible" (p. 138).

There may be drawbacks, however. To the extent that embarrassment is socialized through painful social ridicule as A. H. Buss (1980) suggested, it may actually become too widespread. If trivial transgressions result in huge humiliations, children are likely to develop *exaggerated* fears of social disapproval that may leave them overly sensitive to the evaluations of strangers and overly cautious in their social behavior. In fact, Buss (1980) believed that if children were not jeered for their social mistakes, embarrassment would be much less prevalent; "change the way children are socialized, and embarrassment would be sharply reduced" (p. 233).

As things stand, embarrassment *is* commonplace, and any parent may be grateful for that. Nevertheless, as we'll see in the next chapter, some people grow up with an excessive susceptibility to embarrassment that is rooted in burdensome fears about what others are thinking of them. Some people learn to be too scared of embarrassment, and their socialization may be at fault. If A. H. Buss is correct, we sometimes teach embarrassment with sledgehammers when smaller tools would do the job.

## COGNITIVE DEVELOPMENT

The enforcement of socialized standards begins in earnest (Kopp, 1982), and children become self-aware (Lewis et al., 1989), around age 2. Some of the important influences on the development of embarrassment are thus present rather early in life. There's a third essential component of the developmental process, however, that makes 2-year-olds dramatically different from the adults they will become: They think differently than we do.

The nature and content of a preschooler's thoughts may be hard for us to appreciate. For one thing, young children seem to experience mental activity itself as an episodic, on-and-off endeavor, whereas adults consider a stream of consciousness as a continuous, nonstop operation (Flavell, 1993). There may be times when young children are not much aware of *anything*. Furthermore, the thoughts that a child has will be more single-minded and less complex. Various models of cognitive development all agree that preschoolers have difficulty understanding others' points of view of a given event.

For instance, the famous theorist Jean Piaget held that preschoolers are *egocentric* and self-centered in their thinking; that is, they believe that others see the world as they do, sharing their own wishes and perceptions (Piaget & Inhelder, 1967). Given a choice of silk stockings or a toy truck as a gift for their mothers, 3-year-olds pick the truck, assuming that Mom wants the same thing they do. About half of a group of 5-year-old children will pick the stockings, and all 6-year-olds do (Flavell, Botkin, Fry, Wright, & Jarvis, 1968), but it clearly takes years for a child to recognize that others' perspectives may differ from his or her own. Thus, although toddlers are self-conscious and are developing knowledge about and opinions of themselves, they are not necessarily aware that anyone else may hold other views.

This point was specifically addressed by Robert Selman (1976), who described several levels of perspective taking in children. Selman agreed that preschoolers are egocentric and acknowledged that 6-year-olds may understand that others' thoughts and feelings can be different from their own. However, he argued that 6- and 7-year-olds have difficulty keeping two different perspectives in mind at the same time; they are likely to focus on one or the other, so that discrepancies between multiple perspectives may be hard for them to grasp. In addition, at this age children are still unable to understand fully what others may be thinking of *them*. At 8 and 9 years old, children can better comprehend others' evaluations of themselves, but not until they are 10 or 11 years old, said Selman, are children adept enough to take two points of view simulta-neously; only then are they finally able to compare their own and others' judgments as if they were third-person referees.

The relevance of all this for our understanding of embarrassment is that, to the extent embarrassment is grounded in concern about what others are thinking of us, *it should not take its adult form until young adolescence*, when a person is finally fully able to envision and compre-hend others' judgments of him or her. Of course, this would place the emergence of full-fledged "mature" embarrassment a whole decade after the onset of self-recognition, and would thus be a tad inconsistent with Lewis et al.'s (1989) observation of "embarrassment" in 2-year-olds. Let's see what the data have to say.

First, there is little doubt that "a sea change occurs about 6 or 7 years of age in young children's conception of the causes of emotion" (P. L. Harris, 1993, p. 239). Children's understanding of the sources of emo-tion, their attributions of emotion to others, and their strategies for hiding or expressing emotion all become more subtle and refined with age, and are not completely developed until young adolescence (Saarni & Harris, 1989). For instance, preschoolers deny that people are capable of feeling two different, or "mixed," emotions at the same time, but 10-year-olds readily admit that such feelings are possible (Harter & Whitesell, 1989). In general, then, the development of emotional sophistication goes hand in hand with cognitive development.

Children also become more accustomed to self-conscious emotions as they age. Self-conscious shyness is very rare in 5-year-olds, but is commonplace in 10-year-olds (Crozier & Burnham, 1990). Similarly, 9-year-old children are more familiar with embarrassment than younger children are; in one study, a third of the kindergartners and a fifth of the second-graders could not describe any embarrassing experience, but all of the older children readily could (Seidner, Stipek, & Feshbach, 1988). At 4 years old, children have usually heard the term "embarrassment," but often have no idea what it is (Griffin, 1995). Such findings may mean that preschoolers can experience full-blown embarrassment but simply do not have the verbal skills needed to label it correctly. Never-theless, greater familiarity with embarrassing circumstances also seems to be linked to age, experience, and cognitive development.

More importantly, the nature of the situations that cause childhood embarrassment change as a youngster ages. British researcher Mark Bennett (1989) found that 5- and 8-year-old children were embarrassed by their misdeeds only in the presence of a derisive audience that actively scolded them for their transgressions. If observers reacted to their misbehavior with passivity and silence, no embarrassment occurred; only when an audience clearly communicated its disregard did the children become abashed. In contrast, 11- and 13-year-old children were embarrassed by public transgressions whether observers said anything or not. In a subsequent study, Bennett and Gillingham (1991) showed that *any* response to a predicament from an audience, whether negative or positive (e.g., "Oh dear, poor you! Let me help! I could see it was an accident"), embarrassed most 8-year-olds. Only an obvious rebuke, however, embarrassed 5-year-olds.

Altogether, Bennett's data provide the strongest indication that the development of "mature" embarrassment is a protracted process that depends substantially on role taking and cognitive development. Egocentric preschoolers, who have difficulty understanding others' points of view, were generally unaffected by glaring predicaments unless others made their displeasure known; only in the face of manifest social disapproval did they report any feelings of embarrassment. Third-graders, who are aware of others' evaluations but who still lack sophisticated understanding of them, remained unembarrassed when observers evidenced no reaction to their predicaments, but they became embarrassed when an audience expressed any opinion at all (whether punitive or supportive). Finally, young adolescents, who are capable of complex, adult perspective taking, were embarrassed merely by the knowledge that their predicaments had been witnessed by others. They could apparently be embarrassed by the *assumed* evaluations of others, even in the absence of any overt disregard, and thus exhibited the full-blown, mature embarrassment well known to adults.

The notion that advanced cognitive capabilities are involved in adult embarrassment is consistent with other findings as well. Mature guilt and shame also appear to take years to develop, following a pattern much like that of embarrassment (Ferguson, Stegge, & Damhuis, 1991; Harter & Whitesell, 1989), and children with cognitive impairments such as autism exhibit embarrassments that do *not* fit this developmental course (Capps, Yirmiya, & Sigman, 1992). Overall, the data seem rather clear. Although young children may become embarrassed when they are ridiculed or rebuked, they don't seem to envision other's evaluations readily until they near adolescence, and their embarrassments are limited to those situations in which an audience's displeasure is plain. They may certainly become sheepish and chagrined when they are actively reprimanded by others, but they do not readily become embarrassed by public predicaments that go unmentioned by others until they develop advanced perspective-taking skills.

### "Embarrassment" in Young Children

What *is* going on, then, in a 2-year-old who looks embarrassed in front of a mirror? As you recall, Lewis (1993, 1995) reasoned that early embarrassment comes in two forms—an embarrassment of exposure and an embarrassment of evaluation—that emerge at different ages for largely different reasons. However, the signs of "embarrassment" that accompany self-recognition and that are presumed to reflect an embarrassment of exposure are really not all that prevalent; although it's true that they almost never occur in children who have not become self-conscious, only about a third of children who are self-conscious appear embarrassed when they confront their mirror images (Lewis et al., 1991). Moreover, the prolonged path to "mature" embarrassment I've just described makes other scholars think that the behavior Lewis observed probably wasn't embarrassment at all; for instance, Sharon Griffin (1995, p. 234) argues that Lewis et al.'s (1989) findings indicate "only that children are aware of an audience at this age (without judgmental implications) and experience some emotion (possibly discomfort)" that could be a distant precursor to a mature form of embarrassment.

If you insist on a choice, I have to side with Griffin's view. The data are not conclusive on this point, but I think that it's a bit clumsy to assert that early embarrassment emerges from two discrete pathways, one rooted in exposure and the other in evaluation. It seems more parsimonious to me to suggest that the development of embarrassment is a single continuous process that gradually results in increasingly sophisticated emotion as perspective-taking ability improves. Thus when some 2-year-olds appear coy in response to their reflections I'd not call them embarrassed, at least not in any adult sense of the emotion. They are self-conscious and conspicuous, however, and their sheepish behavior may result from the combined influences of the inborn temperaments that make some children shy (Kagan et al., 1992) and the sheer marvelous novelty of self-recognition.

I'd further disagree with Lewis's assumption that conspicuousness is spontaneously embarrassing to 2-year-olds. Young children are able to blithely commit all sorts of sins without being embarrassed by them, so long as they are not actually punished or criticized for such behavior, so it seems unlikely that mere conspicuousness could cause much chagrin. (Remember my friend who walked downtown in the nude; it didn't trouble her a bit until she was punished for it.) On the other hand, I think that A. H. Buss's (1980) analysis of how conspicuousness—so often associated with negative events—gradually becomes embarrassing is quite plausible.

In any case, despite these small disagreements, it is clear that the embarrassment we know so well as adults is the result of a long, complex process of both maturation and training. Once the capability for embarrassment emerges with self-consciousness, both socialization and cognitive growth seem to provide breadth and depth to our experiences of embarrassment.

## ADOLESCENCE AND BEYOND

The personal foundations for full-fledged embarrassment appear to be in place by the time people enter adolescence. Nevertheless, despite all the socialization one has already encountered, there may be a few new influences on embarrassment in one's teen years. For one thing, adolescents may be able to think like adults but they are just discovering how to act like them. Theorists generally agree that adolescence is a period in which youngsters learn significant new social roles, shape a more complex personal identity, and get blindsided by their newfound sexuality (Waterman, 1982). All of this offers unique potential for embarrassment.

In particular, because their relationships with their peers are becoming more intimate and influential than ever before (Csikszentmihalyi & Larson, 1984),[2] teenagers may be especially concerned with what others are thinking of them. In fact, Arnold Buss (1980) believed that self-conscious social emotions such as embarrassment were more common during the teen years than at any other time. He offered two broad reasons why. First, adolescence brings extraordinary *novelty*; one's body changes dramatically with puberty, drawing attention to remarkable new features of one's physical self. Teens also blunder their way into wholly new social roles, notably in romantic relationships, for which they may feel ill equipped and unprepared. Second, adolescents must cope with unfamiliar *impulses*, both sexual and romantic, that raise compelling new issues of propriety and privacy. Altogether, huge new predicaments must be mastered just as social acceptance and approval become especially consequential. If God wanted to create a perfect recipe for embarrassment, the teen years might be it.

Indeed, adolescents do experience more preoccupation with their public images (Cheek et al., 1986) and stronger fears of blushing (Abe & Masui, 1981) than adults do. When I asked high school students about their recent embarrassments (Miller, 1992), I found that they also report more intense embarrassment, on average, than young adults do. However, they react more strongly to roughly the same events; in keeping with their capacity for "mature" embarrassment, teenagers seem to encounter the same *types* of embarrassment as adults (Sattler, 1965). I found no difference in the frequencies with which high school and college participants experienced the various categories of embarrassment in my 1992 study.

However, younger adolescents may not be quite as likely as older teens or adults to experience some of the more complex events that can be embarrassing. In our "embarrassment diary" study, Cathy Stonehouse and I asked 50 fifth-graders (averaging 11 years old) from two elementary schools in Bryan, Texas, to keep track of their embarrassments for a month (Stonehouse & Miller, 1994). In general, the fifth-graders seemed to encounter simpler, more straightforward embarrassments than college students did. As Table 5.1 shows, more of their embarrassments resulted from individual behavior (nearly all of them from normative public deficiencies) with fewer incidents emerging from transactions with other people. In particular, they reported few interactive predicaments and no bystander incidents at all.

The fifth-graders' distribution of embarrassments was significantly different from that of the collegians, and 11-year-olds may routinely encounter more basic predicaments than adults do. One thing is certain: They definitely get a rougher reception. We asked the youngsters to describe what their audiences said and did once they had become embarrassed, and 53% of the time the onlookers laughed at them or teased them. As we'll see in Chapter 9, this is a much harsher response than adults usually get, and it underlines A. H. Buss's (1980) assumption that, when we're young, others' scrutiny often results in "ridicule, scorn, criticism, or rejection" (p. 243). If these data are typical, it's no wonder that we gradually learn to react sheepishly to conspicuousness and the violation of social rules.

**Table 5.1. Comparing the Embarrassments of College Students and Fifth-Graders**

| Type of embarrassment | Fifth-graders | Collegians |
| --- | --- | --- |
| Individual behavior | 80% | 64% |
| Interactive behavior | 2% | 9% |
| Audience provocation | 18% | 14% |
| Bystander behavior | 0% | 13% |
| | 100% | 100% |

The good news is that our susceptibility to embarrassment probably wanes somewhat during adulthood. No study has yet tracked embarrassment into middle and late adulthood, but all indications point to less frequent and less intense embarrassments after full maturity is attained (Anderson & Kauffman, 1992; Horowitz, 1962). In that sense, then, the development of embarrassment may be a lifelong process. The changes may be less noticeable than in our early years, but our sensitivity to embarrassment and our reactions to our predicaments may continue to evolve throughout our lives.

## CONCLUSIONS

Embarrassment appears to be a "self-conscious" emotion, like pride, shame, and guilt (Tangney & Fischer, 1995), based in the ability to evaluate oneself as a unique person, apart from others. Theorists generally agree that embarrassment requires self-consciousness (e.g., A. H. Buss, 1980), and the earliest signs of anything like embarrassment in young children does coincide with the emergence of self-consciousness during the second or third year. However, self-consciousness may be necessary but not sufficient for embarrassment to occur, because embarrassment seems to require recognition of what *others* are thinking of us, as well. Young children have trouble putting themselves in others' shoes; the fact that others may see things differently than they do does not fully dawn on them until they are 5 or 6 years old. Even then, it may be difficult for them to envision what others are thinking, so they are unlikely to be embarrassed by the possibility of negative evaluations from others unless the audience makes its disapproval plain. Not until they are 10 or 11 do children resemble adults in fretting that others may be judging them negatively in the absence of some clear evidence of disregard.

Children reach this point through the joint influence of cognitive maturation and years of social experience during which they learn shared standards of conduct. It is possible that the prevalence of embarrassment in Western life is due in part to the ready callousness with which observers often react to others' social predicaments. In any case, given the shared impact of self-consciousness, socialization, and cognitive development, it is typical for people to be susceptible to embarrassment as they grow up, although variations in socialization may make some people and some cultures more prone to embarrassment than others. Indeed, it is quite possible for people to differ in their susceptibility to embarrassment, as we will see in the next chapter.

# CHAPTER 6

# *Personality and Culture*

~

If you're like me, you may be less susceptible to embarrassment than you used to be. I haven't formally tracked my "embarrassability" over time, but I'm almost certain that I'm less affected by embarrassing circumstances than I was when I was younger. I seem better able to shrug off my routine pratfalls and cognitive errors without much fuss, accepting them as ordinary examples of the dopey things that happen to everybody. Even real disasters that do get me embarrassed don't elicit as much emotion as they once did.

I think there are several reasons for this. First, I've been studying embarrassment for several years now, and, like anything else that's grown familiar, it has become less fearsome under close inspection. (In fact, by the time you finish this book, I hope that you too will be a bit less embarrassable than you were when you started. I'll try to foster that outcome in Chapter 10.) More importantly, however, I think I've gradually become less worried about what others think of me. With a bit of maturity in my middle age, I've become less self-conscious, so others' evaluations of me are less salient day to day. Moreover, as a college professor, I've made my share of mistakes in front of large audiences, and they rarely turn out as badly as one might expect. Audiences are more forgiving than we often imagine, so there's less to fear than we think. (I'll document this point in Chapter 9.) Altogether, I think that hard-won experience and decreasing dread of others' opinions, combined with a little insight into embarrassment, have gradually made awkward circumstances less threatening to me.

I mention this with two points in mind. On the one hand, it's reassuring to think, if excessive embarrassability is troubling to us, that our susceptibility to embarrassment may change over time. As I mentioned last chapter, concern about others' evaluations is probably at a peak during adolescence, so susceptibility to embarrassment may wane as we gradually become adults. On the other hand, my experiences as a professor and embarrassment researcher have been fairly unique, and you may not have had the chance (like me) to get used to committing cognitive errors in front of 200 people at a time. Moreover, if you're *really* sensitive about what others think of you, you probably wouldn't take a job that gives you a chance to make such obvious public mistakes.

It's likely that our susceptibilities to embarrassment are shaped by our social experiences throughout our lives, and if individuals encounter very different experiences, their openness to embarrassment may differ as well. In addition, to the extent that people *choose* to frequent different social environments, small differences among individuals may be accentuated over time as disparate socialization occurs. Thus, although we can agree on the types of events people find embarrassing (see Chapter 4) and although almost everyone will gradually develop some capacity for embarrassment (Chapter 5), large individual differences in embarrassability can and do exist. They probably result, as the foregoing discussion implies, from the different broad types of *situations* people experience, from stable *personality* differences among people that make them more or less sensitive to embarrassment, and perhaps even from the *interactions* of personalities and situations as different people gravitate to different environments.

This chapter examines these individual differences in embarrassability. As we'll see, some people really are more susceptible to embarrassment than others, and a focus on personality differences will provide a detailed analysis of the personality trait of embarrassability. Then, using a broader situational focus, we'll inquire whether various cultures appear to differ in the way their members experience embarrassment.

## THE TRAIT OF EMBARRASSABILITY

The last chapter described the link between embarrassment and self-consciousness: There are typically no signs of embarrassment in children at all until a capacity for self-consciousness emerges. What I didn't note at the time is that two types of self-consciousness are possible, depending on what one is thinking about. When we attend to our personal, internal feelings, moods, and motives, we are aware of *private* states that are known only to us. In contrast, when we envision how we are being judged by others, our *public* behavior and appearances are more salient. People vary in their chronic tendencies to attend to these two different aspects of themselves and are thus said to differ in their traits of *private self-consciousness* and *public self-consciousness,* respectively (Fenigstein, Scheier, & Buss, 1975). The two tendencies are moderately correlated, so that people who lean toward introspection tend to monitor their public images as well. Nevertheless, a person may be high in one tendency and not in the other, or high in both or neither (A. H. Buss, 1980).

Susceptibility to embarrassment should be mildly related to private self-consciousness because people who are attentive to their moods should be more likely to notice moderate embarrassments. However, if embarrassment really is an emotion that results from concerns about our public images, embarrassability should be even more closely related to public self-consciousness: People who dwell on what others may be thinking of them should be more routinely prone to embarrassment than are people who are usually heedless of what others are thinking.

## The Embarrassability Scale

These are reasonable hypotheses, but testing them would have been difficult had Andre Modigliani (1968) not developed a brief question-naire that ably assesses individual differences in embarrassability. Modigliani created an Embarrassability Scale that contains one-sentence descriptions of 26 potentially embarrassing situations; respondents rate how embarrassed they would be in each of these predicaments, and the sum of their ratings provides an embarrassability score.

The scale was created years ago, but nevertheless contains examples of all the major types of embarrassments detected by recent surveys. It asks about respondents' reactions to normative deficiencies such as public pratfalls and invasions of privacy, awkward interactions caused by a loss of script, audience provocations (such as the singing of "Happy Birthday"), and even bystander predicaments such as empathic embarrassment. Respondents are only imagining how they would be affected by these various events, but, because of the wide range of predicaments included on the scale, most people will be familiar with several of these situations. As a result, people can generate sensible guesses about the extent of their reactions, and, over the 26 items, sizable differences among individuals do emerge.

These differences are meaningful because the scale does predict how people will respond to the actual predicaments they face. In my studies of empathic embarrassment (Miller, 1987), the bystanders' Embarrass-ability Scale scores did significantly forecast how much empathic em-barrassment they would experience when they watched others' predica-ments. Moreover, our surveys of embarrassing circumstances (Miller,

1992; Stonehouse & Miller, 1994) showed that people with higher embarrassability scores really did experience stronger embarrassment when unwanted predicaments occurred. They also became embarrassed more frequently. The scale appears to be valid, tapping real differences among people in susceptibility to day-to-day embarrassment. However, Modigliani (1968) only recruited men for his initial study, and his original version of the scale was written for male respondents. For later studies involving both men and women, I adapted the scale slightly so that it was appropriate for either sex (see Leary, 1991). This updated version of the Embarrassability Scale is shown in Table 6.1.

As you can see, several items still describe situations that apply only to college students (e.g., "Suppose you were alone in an elevator with a professor who had just given you a bad grade"). These can be readily adjusted for other respondents, however (so that the professor becomes, e.g., "a supervisor who gave you a poor evaluation"). If you make such changes and answer the scale yourself, you can compare yourself to the hundreds of collegians who have completed the scale in research studies.

Using the 1-to-5 scale for each item provided in Table 6.1, the average embarrassability score for men is approximately 64. The average score for women is approximately 72 (Miller, 1992, 1995b). The standard deviation for both sexes is close to 14, however, so scores anywhere between 50 and 78 are pretty typical for men, with scores between 58 and 86 being routine for women. Outside those ranges, more extreme scores become increasingly rare.

The difference between the average scores of men and women is statistically significant and usually appears when reactions to embarrassment are measured (Miller, 1995b). For instance, women experience stronger empathic embarrassment than men do (Miller, 1987), and they report recent embarrassments that are more intense (Miller, 1992). Women do not seem to encounter *types* of embarrassment that are any different from those of men; instead, they react more strongly to essentially the same predicaments (Miller, 1992). They may also work harder than men to repair and redress embarrassing circumstances once they have occurred (Gonzales et al., 1990). Importantly, there is substantial variability among the individual embarrassability scores of both men and women, and members of either sex may be either quite susceptible or rather immune to embarrassment. On the whole, however, women are more embarrassable than men.

There may be several reasons why, and I will return to the questions raised by this difference between the sexes in embarrassability. The difference may be more explicable with a fuller understanding of embarrassability itself, however, so let's continue our analysis of the components of the trait for now.

## TABLE 6.1. The Embarrassability Scale

These questions ask whether certain social situations would cause you embarrassment. To be sure that we mean the same thing by "embarrassment," let's say a few words about it. Generally, embarrassment involves feeling self-conscious, awkward, discomforted, or exposed because of the nature of the situation. Remember that you may feel embarrassed for yourself or for someone else. Remember also that mild embarrassment differs considerably from strong embarrassment, while still being a form of embarrassment. Mild embarrassment generally involves a very slight self-consciousness, a mild sensation of awkwardness and uneasiness, and a slight feeling of uncertainty about what to do or say next. On the other hand, strong embarrassment can be extremely unpleasant, involving blushing, fumbling, severe self-consciousness, strong sensations of awkwardness and discomfort, a panicky feeling of being unable to react appropriately to the situation that has been created, and a strong desire to escape the situation and the presence of others.

Read the items below. Try to imagine as vividly as possible that each of these events is happening to you. If they have occurred to you in the past, think back to how you felt at the time. Then, rate how embarrassed you would feel if the event were actually happening to you by using the scale below to describe your reaction:

1 = I would not feel the least embarrassed:
   not awkward or uncomfortable at all.
2 = I would feel slightly embarrassed.
3 = I would feel fairly embarrassed: somewhat self-
   conscious, and rather awkward and uncomfortable.
4 = I would feel quite embarrassed.
5 = I would feel strongly embarrassed: extremely
   self-conscious, awkward, and uncomfortable.

_____ 1. Suppose you were just beginning a talk in front of a class.

_____ 2. Suppose you slipped and fell on a patch of ice in a public place, dropping a bag of groceries.

_____ 3. Suppose you were a dinner guest, and the guest seated next to you spilled his plate on his lap while trying to cut his meat.

_____ 4. Suppose someone stopped you on the street by asking you something, and he turned out to be quite drunk and incoherent.

_____ 5. Suppose a group of friends were singing "Happy Birthday" to you.

_____ 6. Suppose you discovered you were the only person at a particular social occasion without a coat and tie (or dress).

_____ 7. Suppose you were watching an amateur show and one of the performers was trying to do a comedy act, but was unable to make anyone laugh.

_____ 8. Suppose you were calling up a person you had just met for the first time in order to ask him or her for a date.

9. Suppose you were muttering aloud to yourself in an apparently empty room and discovered that someone else was present.

10. Suppose you walked into a bathroom at someone else's house and discovered it was occupied by a member of the opposite sex.

11. Suppose you were watching a play from the audience when it suddenly became clear that one of the actors had forgotten her lines, causing the play to come to a standstill.

12. Suppose you were unable to stop coughing while listening to a lecture.

13. Suppose you were being lavishly complimented on your pleasant personality by your companion on your first date.

14. Suppose you were in a class and you noticed that the teacher had completely neglected to zip his fly.

15. Suppose you entered an apparently empty classroom, turned on the lights, and surprised a couple necking.

16. Suppose you were talking to a stranger who stuttered badly due to a speech impediment.

17. Suppose your mother had come to visit you and was accompanying you to all your classes.

18. Suppose you were a dinner guest and could not eat the main course because you were allergic to it.

19. Suppose you were alone in an elevator with a professor who had just given you a bad grade.

20. Suppose a shabbily dressed man accosted you on the street and asked you for a handout.

21. Suppose you were walking into a room full of people you did not know and were being introduced to the whole group.

22. Suppose you tripped and fell while entering a bus full of people.

23. Suppose you were opening some presents while the donors were sitting around watching.

24. Suppose you asked someone on crutches if he had suffered a skiing accident and he blushed and replied that, no, he was crippled by polio when he was a child.

25. Suppose you had forgotten an appointment with a professor, and remembered it as you met him in the hall the next day.

26. Suppose you were talking in a small group that included a blind student, when someone next to him unthinkingly made a remark about someone being "blind as a bat."

*Note.* Copyright 1968 by Andre Modigliani. Adapted by permission of the author.

## Self-Consciousness and Embarrassability

As it turns out, one's self-consciousness *is* significantly related to one's susceptibility to embarrassment. People who are attentive to their moods and feelings—those who are high in private self-consciousness—are more embarrassable than those who do not tend toward introspection (Leary & Meadows, 1991; Miller, 1995b). This is not an especially strong tendency, however, and there is a stronger connection between public self-consciousness, or attention to one's public image, and embarrassability: People who routinely monitor what others are thinking of them are clearly more susceptible to embarrassment than are those who pay little attention to others' judgments (Edelmann, 1985b; Leary & Meadows, 1991; Miller, 1995b).

This link between public self-consciousness and embarrassability is telling. First, it supports our basic conception of embarrassment as an emotion rooted in our concern for what others may be thinking of us. Second, differences among people in public self-consciousness may also help explain differences among people in reactions to embarrassing circumstances. Bill Froming and his colleagues demonstrated that, with their higher sensitivity to others' evaluations, people high in public self-consciousness were more affected by strangers' judgments of them than were people who were low in public self-consciousness (Froming et al., 1990). Froming et al. invited college students to earn money by singing "The Star Spangled Banner" in front of another student watching from an adjacent room. How long they sang was up to them, but they were paid "by the hour," so the longer their performances, the greater their earnings. Importantly, the person watching them, their audience, was (1) a good friend who knew them well, (2) a complete stranger they would not see again, or (3) a stranger with whom they would discuss the experiment after they were done singing.

You may recall that it's often less embarrassing to do something silly in front of friends than in front of strangers (Chapter 4). Indeed, people low in public self-consciousness sang twice as long for a friend—and for strangers they would not see again—than for someone they did not know whom they would have to face later. Their reactions to this embarrassing situation obviously depended on just who was watching. They were bolder when they could count on continued regard from their audiences (the friends) or simply avoid any feedback from the audiences altogether (the anonymous strangers) than they were when they were likely to hear what the strangers thought of them. In contrast, people high in public self-consciousness did not respond differently to friends than to strangers, and they sang for shorter periods overall. They were eager to avoid the embarrassing task no matter who was watching. In particular, they appeared to care much more than did those low in public self-consciousness about implicit evaluations from a total stranger that they would not soon see again.

One component of embarrassability is thus an elevated sensitivity to evaluations from others. Embarrassable people tend to be high in public self-consciousness and may treat others' judgments as important regardless of who those others are. Less embarrassable people seem to care less about what others may be thinking of them, and they make finer distinctions between the social evaluations that matter and those that do not.

## Social Evaluations and Embarrassability

However, chronic awareness of others' evaluations may not, by itself, be especially risky. Highly embarrassable people also seem to be preoccupied with certain *types* of evaluations from others. Embarrassability is closely linked to another personality characteristic known as *fear of negative evaluation* (Leary & Meadows, 1991; Miller, 1995b), and highly embarrassable people are particularly likely to fear that others may think poorly of them.

People who have a high fear of negative evaluation worry about rejection from others (Leary, 1983). The possibility that others dislike them is rarely far from their minds. In general, they have a chronic dread of others' disregard, and the threat of criticism or derision from others is more salient to them than to those who worry less about others' disdain. Such fear of negative evaluation is related to public self-consciousness (Leary & Meadows, 1991; Miller, 1995b), which makes sense given that one must first be aware of others' evaluations in order to be worried about them. Someone can be high in public self-consciousness without worrying overmuch about others' scorn, however, so the two do not necessarily go hand in hand.

I studied the relationships among public self-consciousness, fear of negative evaluation, and embarrassability by asking 310 collegians to complete scales measuring the three traits (Miller, 1995b). Susceptibility to embarrassment was more closely linked to fear of negative evaluation than to public self-consciousness per se. Moreover, fear of negative evaluation was a better predictor of high embarrassability; that is, I learned more about the extent of a person's embarrassability by measuring his or her fear of negative evaluation than by assessing public self-consciousness. In a sense, embarrassability was characterized by a certain kind of aversive self-consciousness: Embarrassable people were aware of what others might be thinking of them, but they also tended to worry that others' judgments were negative and undesirable.

Other traits that are linked to embarrassability also fit this pattern. Modigliani (1968) found that embarrassability was related to feelings of social inadequacy, so that people who felt relatively unloved and unlovable were more susceptible to embarrassment. Mark Leary and Sarah Meadows (1991) showed that embarrassability was linked both to the extent of one's desire to avoid rejection from others and to concern about one's public physical appearance. I found that embarrassability was associated both with the desire to win acceptance and approval from others and with a lack of self-confidence in social situations (Miller, 1995b). These findings all suggest that highly embarrassable people wish to receive favorable evaluations from others but doubt that they can. As Modigliani suggested when he developed the Embarrassability Scale, "greater embarrassability is a result of the *simultaneous presence* of two traits: (1) a sensitivity to the immediate evaluations of others, and (2) a general readiness to believe that these evaluations are more negative than they really are" (1968, p. 325).

This pattern puts highly embarrassable people between a rock and a hard place. They are especially attentive to what others think of them, but they dread such evaluations and anticipate disapproval from others. Is there a clear reason why? Perhaps embarrassable people are clumsy, inept folks who justifiably fear negative evaluation because they often make mistakes and bear the brunt of others' disregard. In fact, my study of embarrassability (Miller, 1995b) specifically examined this possibility.

## Embarrassability and Social Skill

Arnold Buss (1980) surmised that social skill should affect one's susceptibility to embarrassment. He argued that

> people who are socially clumsy tend to blurt out statements that should not be said, to call people by wrong names, to lack poise and polish in their interactions with others. Lacking social skills, they repeatedly make the small mistakes that cause them to feel foolish, silly, uncomfortable—in a word, embarrassed. (p. 141)

This sounds plausible, but it's important to specify what we're talking about when we study "social skill." Modern conceptions of social skill stress that it is best studied as a collection of discrete but interrelated talents that combine to produce a person's global level of social competence. For instance, Brian Spitzberg and Bill Cupach (1989) identified two fundamental features of competent interactive behavior. They noted that one basic element of social skill is "effectiveness," the ability to regulate and control one's behavior with skill and grace; this notion of interpersonal dexterity and deftness may be what most people think of as "social skill." However, another key component of skillful behavior is "appropriateness," the ability to recognize and adhere to important norms and expectations. In order to do the right thing, people have to be sensitive and astute enough to know what it is. Adroit interaction is both effective *and* appropriate, and embarrassment may presumably result from deficiencies of either type.

Social skill, then, is multifaceted. With this in mind, I measured these talents with a Social Skill Inventory created by Ron Riggio (1986) that assesses six different aspects of interpersonal competence (Miller, 1995b). In particular, Riggio's inventory examines both the effectiveness and appropriateness of both verbal and nonverbal social behavior. Individuals' abilities to regulate their own facial expressions are measured, as is the dexterity with which they make small talk and manage their interactions. Both the ability to read others' emotions and astuteness in judging others' expectations in a given situation are also assessed. In addition, the inventory yields a total score that combines these separate talents and is indicative of general social competence.

Interestingly, susceptibility to embarrassment was not related at all to the level of one's global social skill. It's fair to say that people who, on the whole, have poor social skill are not more prone to embarrassment than are people who are much more skillful. All by itself, that result puts embarrassability in a different class from social anxieties such as shyness or stage fright, because such anxieties *are* significantly associated with generally poor skills (Leary & Kowalski, 1995). For instance, I found a sizable relationship between total skills and shyness that showed that inept people were much more likely to be shy than were those who were more adept at interaction (Miller, 1995b). People of lower social competence are evidently more likely to be apprehensive and inhibited—that is, shy—*before* anything goes wrong with their interactions, but do not necessarily tend to react more strongly (with embarrassment) *after* some predicament occurs. Conversely, high global social skill apparently does not make someone less susceptible to embarrassment; given the diversity of the pitfalls that can cause us embarrassment (and given that some embarrassments are not of our making), people with generally good skills can be embarrassed just like everybody else.

It would be misleading to stop with that conclusion, however, because certain *components* of social skill identified by Riggio's (1986) inventory *were* linked to embarrassability. People who were proficient at controlling their interactive behavior did tend to be less prone to embarrassment than were people who were less socially deft and dexterous. To a lesser degree, people who were good at managing their emotional expressions, who could look unruffled even when they weren't, were also less embarrassable. The "effectiveness" of a person's social behavior, then, did say something about how embarrassable that person was likely to be. Presumably, such talents both help one avoid predicaments that befall others who are less able (as A. H. Buss, 1980, predicted), and help one repair unavoidable predicaments with a minimum of fuss.

However, a different kind of skill was even more closely related to embarrassability. The single best predictor of how embarrassable a person was likely to be was that person's sensitivity to social norms. Awareness of, and concern about, the normative appropriateness of one's behavior was linked to greater susceptibility to embarrassment. Embarrassable people were especially attentive to social rules, they dreaded any violation of them, and they expected more negative consequences when any transgression occurred. In comparison, people low in embarrassability took a more relaxed view of social norms; they paid less attention to them and were less apprehensive when a norm was broken.

Now, it's clear that the ability to understand the expectations of others and to discern what one must do to behave properly in a given situation is an adaptive, valuable skill. A visiting diplomat does well, for instance, when she can quickly judge how best to honor her hosts. A job applicant may be more successful when his jokes fit the occasion than when they do not. However, too much of a good thing is not necessarily desirable; an excessive concern about social appropriateness may leave one at undue risk when predicaments occur. Moreover, a person who is especially strict about appropriate behavior may not only find a given transgression to be more fearsome, there may be more events to fear; such a person may be beset with worry over small difficulties that others find unremarkable. In fact, our studies of embarrassing circumstances did show that highly embarrassable people do not encounter different types of embarrassment than anyone else, they just encounter them more often and react more strongly to the same sorts of predicaments when they do occur (Miller, 1992; Stonehouse & Miller, 1994). In particular, we found that people who were more attentive to social norms—and those with higher fear of negative evaluation—suffered more frequent and more intense embarrassments than did those who were less attentive or fearful.

Thus, it appears that, to some degree, clumsy, maladroit people may be more embarrassable than the rest of us because their behavior is less effective and they blunder into more predicaments. Arnold Buss's (1980) hypothesis that graceless people should be more susceptible to embarrassment is true, to a limited extent. A larger component of embarrassability, however, is an exaggerated attentiveness to and concern about the appropriateness of one's behavior. Highly embarrassable people wish to do the right thing and to be accepted by others, and these motives lead them both to notice and to dread violations of social rules more than others do. They are attuned to others' expectations, and are more likely to recognize any departures from a given norm of conduct. They are also less tolerant of such violations when they occur (as they inevitably do). Their reactions of chagrin and abashment are more intense—in part because they routinely worry that others are judging them negatively— and they are likely to overestimate the current damage being done. Whatever their other social skills, they (1) hold themselves to stricter, less forgiving codes of conduct; and (2) chronically worry about what others are thinking of them, more than the rest of us do.

## Embarrassability and Neuroticism

One gets the feeling that excessive embarrassability is an undesirable liability. At the extreme, highly embarrassable people are likely to be unnecessarily nervous, exhibiting exaggerated dread of others' judgments and overreacting to the ordinary peccadillos of social life. They may be edgy, always expecting the worst, and their emotions may be more labile, as they become flustered by situations most of us ignore or shrug off. Thus it may not be surprising that there is a tendency for highly embarrassable people to be more neurotic, too. *Neuroticism* describes a person's proclivity toward worry and sudden, anxious shifts in arousal, and there is a link of small-to-moderate size between neuroticism and embarrassability (Edelmann & McCusker, 1986; Kelly, 1994; see also Darvill, Johnson, & Danko, 1992).

Obviously, some susceptibility to embarrassment is normal. More-over, given the developmental processes that help create it (Chapter 5), it may be unavoidable. When people come to be highly embarrassable, however, they also display other traits that may make them characteristically moody, unhappy people.

## Sex Differences in Embarrassability

Portraying excessive embarrassability in a negative light makes it treacherous to return now to some speculation about why women are more embarrassable than men. Let me remind you, though, that the average difference between the sexes is rather small compared to the range of embarrassability among members of each sex. Either men or women may be very high or quite low in susceptibility to embarrassment, and the differences between high and low scorers (of either sex) are much, much greater than the difference between the sexes. It's a clear mistake to think of women as generally high in embarrassability and men as generally low, because that simply isn't true. Nevertheless, there is a measurable, reliable difference between the sexes, on average, that begs for explanation.

The first thing I should note is that there's nothing unique about the sex difference in embarrassability. Women generally tend to experience stronger emotions than men, so that "more strongly felt and more volatile emotions" are characteristic of women throughout their lives (Brody & Hall, 1993, p. 449; see also Fujita, Diener, & Sandvik, 1991, but cf. LaFrance & Banaji, 1992). In particular, women consistently experience stronger negative emotions about themselves such as shame (Stapley & Haviland, 1989), guilt (Tangney, 1990), and, of course, embarrassment (Miller, 1992).

One possible reason why women's emotions are more intense is that people *expect* them to be stronger. Many cultures share stereotypes that portray men as more stoic than women (Ruble, 1983), and these beliefs can influence what individuals think about their own emotions. Michele Grossman and Wendy Wood (1993) found that men's and women's accounts of their emotions were correlated with their broader beliefs about sex differences in emotion; those who accepted the cultural expectation that women were more emotional than men reported personal experiences that more closely fit that pattern than did those who did not share that expectation. Grossman and Wood also obtained physiological data indicating that, regardless of their expectations, women reacted more strongly to negative emotional situations than did men, so that real—as well as reported—differences in emotion do exist between the sexes. Nonetheless, the belief that women are ordinarily more emotional than men is widespread, and it may not be an innocent assumption. Such a belief can set in motion real events that shape men's and women's emotions differently.

For instance, parents who subscribe to the stereotype may discuss emotions more fully with their daughters than their sons, display a wider range of emotion to their daughters, and allow richer expressions of emotion from their daughters than from their sons (Brody & Hall, 1993). Over time, very different socialization pressures may train young men and women to experience emotion to different degrees.

In addition, there may be other influences that make it especially likely that women will experience emotions rooted in social evaluation—such as embarrassment—more intensely. More often than men, women may find themselves in situations in which it is important to maintain the good will of their associates. As children, girls play in small, collaborative groups more often than boys, whose play, in contrast, is characterized by competition, conflict, and one-upmanship (Maccoby, 1990). Girls' entertainments are more dependent on cooperation and consensus, and, as a result, girls may ordinarily be more concerned than boys with maintaining the approval and acceptance of their peers. Boys' play may also involve more teasing, ridicule, and intentional embarrassment than girls ordinarily encounter, so that boys may have more experience at surviving unwanted predicaments (Leary & Kowalski, 1995). For various reasons, then, the threat of disapproval or rejection may affect girls more, arousing stronger reactions when social censure becomes salient and making them more susceptible to embarrassment.

Thereafter, as adults, prevailing social norms may often place women in positions of lower power than those traditionally occupied by men (so that, for instance, they receive less pay for similar work and are more likely to be supervised by men than to supervise men themselves; see Eagly, 1987). As typical subordinates, women may often be more dependent on others than men are, and may thus have more reason to fear social disapproval: Rejection from others may ordinarily be more costly for women, entailing greater material, as well as psychological, losses. Stronger concern over the acceptability of their behavior would then be justifiable, and social transgressions more fearsome. Higher embarrassability would result.

In fact, for whatever reason, women do display higher fears of negative evaluation and stronger motives to avoid rejection from others than men do (Miller, 1995b). They also possess better skill at nonverbal communication, which may simply add fuel to the fire. Women tend to interpret others' emotional expressions more accurately than men do (Hall, 1984; Riggio, 1986), and may thus be able to recognize subtle signs of disapproval from others that escape some men entirely. Given similar social predicaments, perceptive women may become more embarrassed than others because they are more astutely aware of just how bad things really are!

It's even possible that women's emotions are affected more by external, social events than men's are. James Pennebaker and Tomi-Ann Roberts (1992) suggested that men are more likely than women to detect accurately and then rely on their own internal, visceral cues to decide what they are feeling. In comparison, according to Pennebaker and Roberts, women's emotions are more likely than men's to be influenced by the situations and circumstances around them. Thus, when external events are dramatic and compelling, as embarrassing predicaments often are, we should not be surprised to find women reacting more strongly.

All of these explanations are possible and they all may actually be true, because they are not mutually exclusive or incompatible and each is consistent with the available data. They all remain speculative, however, so I'll not assert a preference for any one of them. Nevertheless, collectively, they are sound reminders that susceptibility to embarrassment may spring from several sources, and few, if any, of us are immune. People may vary in their concern about others' evaluations for diverse reasons, and meaningful differences in embarrassability exist. Nevertheless, it is normal for people to care what others are thinking of them, and it is certainly normal to be embarrassable.

## EMBARRASSMENT ACROSS CULTURES

In fact, embarrassment occurs around the world, in Eastern as well as Western cultures. Embarrassment has been observed among Africans, Samoans, and the Balinese (Eibl-Eibesfelt, 1972), and researchers have studied embarrassment in the United Kingdom, Greece, Italy, Spain, and West Germany (Edelmann et al., 1989); Iran (Hashimoto & Shimizu, 1988); and Japan (Cupach & Imahori, 1993; Edelmann & Iwawaki, 1987; Sueda & Wiseman, 1992). The message that emerges from these investigations is clear: There is notable similarity in embarrassment across cultures. Regardless of their language, religion, climate, or level of industrialization (to name a few cultural variables), people suffer embarrassment when unwanted events reveal undesired information about themselves to others.

For example, one international group of scholars found that adolescents in Sweden, Hungary, India, and Yemen could all produce examples of embarrassing predicaments when asked, and all four groups of youngsters found such events similarly aversive (Stattin, Magnusson, Olah, Kassin, & Reddy, 1991). In another investigation, Hashimoto and Shimizu (1988) found that Iranian children agreed rather closely with Japanese children about the embarrassing potential of such predicaments as "falling off your bicycle" and "opening the toilet door and finding someone inside." Bill Cupach and Todd Imahori (1993) asked college students in Illinois and in western Japan to describe a past embarrassment that had been caused by someone else, and found that similar types of audience provocation, team embarrassment, and empathic embarrassment occurred with similar frequencies in the two groups. Around the globe, people care what others think of them (Stattin et al., 1991), and embarrassment appears to be much like other emotions in resulting from antecedent events that vary little from culture to culture (see Matsumoto, Kudoh, Scherer, & Wallbott, 1988; Mesquita & Frijda, 1992). Remarkably, the events that caused your last embarrassment may also have troubled others who will not be able to read this book until it is translated into their language!

This is not to say, however, that others elsewhere would have *responded* as you did when you were last embarrassed. Because there are robust differences across cultures in the norms that govern expressions of emotion (Ekman, 1972), cultures do differ in the extent to which their peoples will try to suppress or regulate an emotion once it occurs (Matsumoto et al., 1988; Scherer & Wallbott, 1994). Thus, although embarrassment results from similar events and likely *feels* the same— causing similar physiological responses—around the world (Edelmann, 1990b), there appear to be subtle variations among cultures in the typical nonverbal behaviors that accompany embarrassment (Edelmann et al., 1989) and larger differences in the strategies with which people will ordinarily try to cope with embarrassment once it has occurred (Cupach & Imahori, 1993; Sueda & Wiseman, 1992). In particular—as our discussion of responses to embarrassment in Chapter 9 will show— North Americans and Japanese may respond somewhat differently to the same predicament. Embarrassment seems to spring from similar sources across the globe, but specific cultural norms can have much to do with how it is managed and expressed.

Moreover, a culture's norms can gradually *change* over time, so there can also be differences in the embarrassing potential of a given event from generation to generation within a given culture. A close reading of American advice columnists such as Ann Landers over the past 40 years will show that behavior that was once routinely embarrassing— such as breast-feeding a baby in public, no matter how discreetly it was done—can slowly become unremarkable. In fact, I know of a woman in her late 50s who, as a young woman, used to be routinely abashed to be seen in public when she was visibly pregnant. She remembers this wryly, because she would feel no such chagrin today. Obviously, the standards with which we judge desirable conduct are continuously evolving, and embarrassments we take for granted may ultimately be much less troubling to our grandchildren.

## Embarrassability and Culture

Another important difference among cultures is more subtle, but perhaps more fundamental. A culture's basic assumptions about an individual's connections to others may help make its people generally more or less susceptible to embarrassment in the first place. We have seen that embarrassability is closely tied to a person's concerns about what others are thinking of him or her, and, as we noted just now, such concerns are universal (Stattin et al., 1991). What varies from culture to culture is the concept of the self that is being judged by others.

Western cultures such as the United States tend to foster "individualism," a perspective that encourages their members to think of themselves as unique, independent individuals who are responsible for their own behavior. In contrast, Eastern cultures tend to support "collectivism," a view that stresses a person's interrelatedness with and accountability to others (Markus & Kitayama, 1991). Whereas members of individualistic cultures celebrate their autonomy and guide their actions with personal, idiosyncratic attitudes and ideals, members of collectivistic cultures emphasize their family and group memberships and stress the importance of shared norms and duties as guides to personal conduct (Triandis, 1994). Higher value is placed on conformity and harmony with others in collectivistic cultures than in individualistic ones.

At the personal level, Theodore Singelis and William Sharkey (1995) have argued that these cultural ideologies result in rather different patterns of self-construal, which they describe as "independent" and "interdependent" conceptions of self. Broadly, independence is tied to self-reliance and needs for uniqueness whereas interdependence is associated with concern for others and belonging. When Singelis and Sharkey developed scales to measure these two aspects of self-construal, they found that Asian Americans at the University of Hawaii had more interdependent and less independent conceptions of themselves than European Americans did. People with roots in collectivistic cultures had relatively interdependent self-concepts, whereas those from individualistic backgrounds had more independent conceptions of self.

Interestingly, the Asian American students, who had roots in China, Japan, Korea, or the Philippines, were more embarrassable, on average, than the European Americans were. Given the same predicaments, people with Eastern backgrounds expected to feel stronger embarrassment than that experienced by those from Western cultures. Edelmann and Iwawaki (1987) also observed this effect in Japanese adults and found that their embarrassments tended to last longer, too. Evidently, cultures that stress group harmony and collective, as opposed to individual, honor and respectability tend to imbue their members with more embarrassability than do cultures in which prestige and virtue are matters of individual, rather than group, conduct. One's interrelatedness with others is more salient in a collectivistic culture than in an individualistic one, and one's misdeeds reflect on others to a greater extent. Thus there is more to be embarrassed about when one misbehaves in a collectivistic culture; one's actions can more readily embarrass others as well as oneself.

However, Singelis and Sharkey (1995) also determined that a person's type of self-construal was a better predictor of his or her embarrassability than was his or her country of origin. The independence and interdependence of the individuals within a cultural group varied, and embarrassability was more closely related to these variables than to culture per se. In particular, although interdependent self-construals were common among Asian Americans, they occurred often in European Americans as well. Here, then, is another personality trait that helps describe a person's susceptibility to embarrassment; anyone who especially values his or her family ties, or who thinks of him- or herself as a team player rather than a rugged individualist, may be more embarrassable than someone who does not.

Certain cultures seem to make such self-concepts more likely and may thus be relatively "embarrassment prone." Such cultural differences are not especially dramatic: Embarrassment really does seem to be a human universal (e.g., Eibl-Eibesfeldt, 1972, 1989), and the differences in embarrassability that exist among cultures are quite small compared to the differences that exist among the individuals within a given culture. Still, it is intriguing that by generally orienting us toward either individuality or belongingness, broad, unspoken cultural perspectives may help make us more or less embarrassable than we otherwise might be. Our personal susceptibilities to embarrassment clearly result from our idiosyncratic personalities and skills, but our cultures may supply a world view that plays a recognizable part as well.

## CONCLUSIONS

Embarrassability varies widely from person to person and, to a lesser extent, from culture to culture. The deftness and dexterity with which a person interacts with others is important because skilled people are less embarrassable than are those who are less adept. Even more telling, however, is a person's concern for what others may be thinking of him or her. People who are especially attentive to social norms and who particularly dread the disapproval that can result from breaking those norms react more strongly to social predicaments than do those who heed others' opinions less (Miller, 1995b). Collectivistic societies emphasize shared norms and a person's links to others, and thus may make their members somewhat more embarrassable than individualistic cultures do (Singelis & Sharkey, 1995).

Nevertheless, embarrassment appears to be pandemic, resulting from reasonably similar events worldwide (e.g., Cupach & Imahori, 1993). This in itself is remarkable and establishes one of the fundamental conditions that allow us to consider embarrassment a basic human emotion (Ekman, 1992). However, although I have described the events that cause embarrassment (Chapter 4) and have now detailed the personalities that are most susceptible to them, I have not yet examined *why* embarrassment occurs at all. What is it exactly about a predicament that causes embarrassment?

This is an essential question, and I'm a bit embarrassed it's taken me this long to get to it. I've delayed consideration of this issue by design, however; I believed that an analysis of the central cause of embarrassment would make more sense after a survey of developmental processes, embarrassing circumstances, and embarrassability was complete. As we'll see in the next chapter, each of those areas of inquiry bears on a search for the fundamental source of embarrassment.

CHAPTER 7

# The Causes
# of Embarrassment

∽

Years ago, when I began to study embarrassment in earnest, I was usually reluctant to tell new acquaintances exactly what my research specialty was. People often seemed to think that embarrassment was a "cute" topic that was frivolous or trivial, and, although I found it fascinating, I had to admit that it was an uncommon topic with uncertain applications. I sometimes felt like apologizing for my "odd" interest.

There's no question that those days are past. Our understanding of embarrassment is much richer now, and I can justifiably assert that studies of embarrassment bear on central components of social interaction. By examining how our transactions can fail, embarrassment research helps illuminate the basic workings of our interchanges with others, mechanisms that structure our daily lives. Even more importantly, embarrassment speaks to our fundamental natures as social animals. The very existence and prevalence of embarrassment speaks volumes about the nature of humanity.

Now these are bold declarations, but I think they are supportable. Our task in this chapter is to question *why* embarrassment occurs. As we will see, the answer hinges on just what it is that is troubling about embarrassing predicaments, and that, in turn, points to vital human motivations that drive interaction and delineate our species. I'll begin by introducing the basic component of interaction from which embarrassment springs.

## IMPRESSION MANAGEMENT

The way we are treated by others typically depends on what those others think of us, and because of this, whether or not we are consciously aware of it, we often try to influence the impressions of us that others form. This process of trying to control how we are perceived by others is called "self-presentation" or *impression management* (Leary & Kowalski, 1990), and it is "a central part of the very nature of social interaction" (Schlenker, 1980, p. 7).

Almost everything people do in public may be strategically regulated in the service of impression management. When they are deliberately trying to make a certain impression, people may carefully choose their apparel and edit what they say about themselves (Zanna & Pack, 1975), adjust their nonverbal behavior (Leary, 1995), and even decide how much to eat (Pliner & Chaiken, 1990). In public restrooms, people are more likely to wash their hands when others are present than when they are alone (Pedersen, Keithly, & Brady, 1986), and college students are more likely to wear school insignia to class when their football teams are winning than when their teams are losing (Cialdini et al., 1976). Both of these are small instances of impression management; people like to publicize their associations with winners and demonstrate their decorum, but they may not go to the trouble if no one is around to be impressed.

On very rare occasions, such behavior is manipulative and deceptive, and people pretend to be things they are not. Most of the time, however, impression management is appropriate, healthy, and adaptive (Leary, 1995). It communicates to others what we wish them to know about us, and that ordinarily emerges from the real self-images we actually possess. The information we disclose is edited, of course, but it usually conveys an accurate (if incomplete) image of who we really are. Impression management thus increases the chances that we will be perceived as we wish *and* deserve to be, and allows interaction to proceed with less confusion and greater grace.

Not all impression management is planned, and no one would suggest that people are always conscious of how they want to impress others next. To the contrary, when a person succeeds in creating a desired public image to which he or she is entitled, patterns of behavior consistent with that image can become personal habits of public presentation that are quite nonconscious (Schlenker, 1980). Such behaviors become routine by being both advantageous and correct. The person provides a coherent persona that gives others a reasonable idea of what to expect from him or her, and, because the person can fulfill those expectations, interaction proceeds smoothly and efficiently.

The processes of impression management are now widely acknowledged to be "a ubiquitous feature of social behavior" (Schlenker & Weigold, 1992, p. 136) that lie "at the heart of interpersonal processes" (p. 134), but this has not always been so. Back in the 1950s, sociologist Erving Goffman, who began the scientific study of embarrassment, was also the first to describe this aspect of social interaction in detail. In a ground-breaking book, *The Presentation of Self in Everyday Life*, Goffman (1959) eloquently compared social behavior to a theatrical performance in which actors played parts complete with scripts, props, and backstage areas where the actors could relax and drop their roles.

As in any theatrical play, an interaction could be disrupted by people flubbing their lines or acting out of character, and for Goffman, a central goal in interaction was the creation and maintenance of a "face," or coherent character, that would allow a person to play a predictable part in the theater of life. A person was

> said to *have,* or *be in,* or *maintain* face when . . . [the behavior he displays] presents an image of him that is internally consistent, that is supported by judgments and evidence conveyed by other participants, and that is confirmed by evidence conveyed through impersonal agencies in the situation. (Goffman, 1955, p. 214)

A consistent, dependable face was vital; without it, one's coactors would not know what to expect, everyone's performance would suffer, and interaction would break down.

Thus, predictable, proficient interaction was thought to depend on participants' abilities to construct and maintain comprehensible, coherent public images. Any uncertainty was unsettling. An inconsistency in an actor's smooth impression management could leave everyone at a loss; Goffman (1959, p. 51) observed that "even sympathetic audiences can be momentarily disturbed, shocked, and weakened in their faith by the discovery of a picayune discrepancy in the impressions presented to them." It was at such moments, Goffman believed, when unwanted events provided undesired information to one's audience, that *embarrassment* occurred. For Goffman, the flustered chagrin of embarrassment was likely when a person realized that "the expressive facts at hand threaten or discredit the assumptions a participant finds he has projected about his identity" (1956, p. 269). Embarrassment thus resulted from acute failures of impression management that endangered one's public "performances."

This perspective on embarrassment has influenced almost every analysis of the state conducted since Goffman's time. His rich descriptions of flustered actors and audiences trying to regain their poise and reestablish their scripts drew attention to unstudied phenomena and helped prompt the first empirical studies of embarrassment in the 1960s. Goffman was, in many respects, the progenitor of modern embarrassment research.

However, Goffman did not elaborate exactly what it was about these aversive breaches of information that caused an emotional response. He cleverly described the arousal and incapacitation that could accompany embarrassment but did not specify why failures of impression management should have such effects. Consideration of the fundamental root of embarrassment has fallen to more recent theorists, who have generated four different views of why embarrassment occurs.

## POSSIBLE CAUSES OF EMBARRASSMENT

Three of the modern models of embarrassment follow very closely from Goffman's theatrical perspective, and one of them even takes its name from Goffman's approach.

### The Dramaturgic Model

Maury Silver, John Sabini, and Jerry Parrott (1987) suggested that embarrassment occurs because fumbled public performances are intrinsically aversive. Unwanted predicaments disrupt one's script and disorder one's expectations; interaction becomes more awkward and clumsy when an actor or audience has to attend to an embarrassing interruption. For Silver and his colleagues, embarrassment is the flustered uncertainty that follows a failure of impression management that leaves a person at a loss about what to do or say next. The agitation and aversive arousal of embarrassment occur when a person suddenly realizes that he or she is unable to calmly and gracefully continue a performance.

Silver et al. (1987) acknowledged that embarrassed people are often worried about what other people are thinking of them, but they averred that problems with one's public image merely accompany, and do not *cause*, embarrassment. They suggested that, "the unpleasantness of embarrassment often, *but not necessarily*, stems from the loss of esteem [in others' eyes]. The only source of unpleasantness that *necessarily* accompanies embarrassment is flustering caused by the perception that there is no character that one can coherently perform" (p. 51). Thus, for Silver et al., the primary reason that embarrassed people feel "flustered, confused, or stymied" (p. 50) is because of their "inability to act a part" (p. 53).

This emphasis on sudden dramaturgical inadequacy fits the feelings of embarrassment pretty well. Most people do feel awkward, inept, and immobilized when they are embarrassed (Parrott & Smith, 1991; Sattler, 1963). Still, do people freeze up just because something unexpected happens and it's hard to adjust, or is there another influence at work as well?

## The Social Evaluation Model

Another view holds that, instead of awkward uncertainty, the active ingredient in embarrassment is concern for what others are thinking of us. In this model, failures of impression management are aversive because they lead audiences to form undesired impressions, and it is these evaluations that people fear most. The predominant cause of the physical and psychological arousal of embarrassment is believed to be the acute threat of unwanted social evaluation that accompanies public predicaments (e.g., Edelmann, 1987; Manstead & Semin, 1981).

The social evaluation perspective acknowledges that embarrassing predicaments often leave one at a loss for what to do and say next. However, such awkwardness is thought to be as much a *result* of one's embarrassment as a cause of it. Uncertainty and a clueless loss of poise in response to a predicament can certainly exacerbate one's embarrassment, in this view, but they do so primarily because they further jeopardize one's endangered social image, not because they are so aversive themselves.

Importantly, the social evaluation model holds that *any* potential evaluation that suggests that an undesired impression has been made on an audience can cause embarrassment. Negative evaluations are usually embarrassing because we typically want to be liked and respected by others. Nevertheless, if one wants to be disliked—by wanting to seem intimidating and fearsome, for example—positive evaluations such as acceptance and approval may actually cause chagrin. Envision a macho gang member being complimented on his tattoos by an elderly woman he passes on the street; if he wants to project an image of dangerousness, a modest compliment from someone who seems unafraid might be quite embarrassing. Thus, the social evaluation perspective does not assume that people always seek to elicit favorable (or socially desirable) judgments from others; it merely asserts that people want to avoid evaluations that would indicate that their attempts to construct a desired image have failed.

The social evaluation model thus posits a more central role for public self-consciousness in the origins of embarrassment than the dramaturgic model does. This perspective assumes that one must be concerned about others' opinions of oneself in order to be embarrassed;

presumably, if a person cares not at all what others think, he or she should be immune to embarrassment (at least in front of that particular audience). In contrast, the dramaturgic model argues that, although one must be aware of others' judgments in order to be motivated to engage in impression management, the severity of one's embarrassment depends on the extent of one's indecisiveness and uncertainty in response to a predicament rather than on one's concern about what others may be thinking.

The social evaluation model is popular among embarrassment researchers (see Edelmann, 1987), but even those who accept most of its assumptions don't necessarily agree that concern about others' opinions is the bedrock of embarrassment. Instead, according to a third view of embarrassment, negative social evaluations simply set in motion the further events that actually cause embarrassment. Andre Modigliani, the creator of the Embarrassability Scale, is one who holds this view.

## Situational Self-Esteem

Modigliani (1971, p. 16) agreed that "embarrassment reflects a failure in one's self-presentation *to others*," and noted that embarrassed people are typically mortified by the realization that their "ineptness will be observed and negatively evaluated by others." However, he believed that the root cause of embarrassment was a temporary loss of self-esteem that resulted from such public failures. In particular, the knowledge that others may be negatively judging a poor public performance was thought to lead to a "special, short-lived, but often acute, loss of self-esteem" (p. 16) based in disregard from the current audience. Because the disapproval of oneself that causes embarrassment is tied to a specific predicament that is limited in duration (unlike the chronic disapproval that accompanies global low self-esteem), Modigliani suggested that embarrassment stems from a loss of *situational self-esteem*.

Thus, for Modigliani, negative social evaluations do not cause embarrassment all by themselves. Instead, they lead one to judge oneself badly, and it is a person's own private disapproval of his or her public acts that produces embarrassment. From this perspective, it would presumably be hard to embarrass a person who remains steadfastly sure of him- or herself despite an inept performance that elicits clear disapproval from important others. No matter what unwelcome surprises occurred, no matter what others were known to be thinking, a person who retained a positive self-evaluation would remain unembarrassed.

A similar assumption underlies the fourth and final model of embarrassment. According to this view, however, embarrassment does not result from failed impression management at all. Instead, it stems from the negative arousal that follows violations of one's personal standards for one's own conduct.

## The Personal Standards Model

Mary Babcock (1988) proposed that embarrassment occurs when a person realizes that his or her behavior is in some way inconsistent with his or her idiosyncratic ideals. Babcock suggested that each of us has an individual "persona" that is characterized by the attitudes, values, and abilities that are most important to us. These combine to form personal guides to conduct that "can be thought of as a set of rules or guidelines that specify how that particular individual should act in a given situation" (Babcock & Sabini, 1990, p. 154). The emotional arousal of embarrassment occurs, according to Babcock, when one becomes aware of a discrepancy between one's actions and one's current standards of behavior (see Higgins, 1989, for a similar view of the origins of emotion).

Babcock (1988) acknowledged that when others are aware of our actions, behavior that would violate our own standards usually creates a threat of unwanted social evaluation as well. However, the more distressing component of a typical predicament, she asserted, is our painful personal knowledge of our shortcomings. Thus, with this perspective, an event should not be embarrassing—no matter how outrageous one's behavior seems to others—if one's actions are acceptable to oneself. On the other hand, embarrassment should routinely result from private misbehavior that occurs when no one else is present; the only necessary condition for embarrassment is undesired behavior that departs from our self-imposed standards, even if it is known to no one but ourselves.

## SIFTING THROUGH THE POSSIBILITIES

Although these four models of embarrassment all propose different phenomena as the ultimate cause of embarrassment, they are not mutually exclusive, and each may contain an important grain of truth. Many different events can cause a degree of embarrassment, and (1) an awkward loss of script, (2) the fear of unwanted social evaluations, (3) a circumscribed blow to your sense of self-worth, and (4) the painful realization that you have just failed yourself may each cause certain types of embarrassment. Furthermore, many embarrassments undoubtedly contain all four components, so that all four phenomena may contribute to our emotional response to some predicaments (Harré & Parrott, 1996).

On the other hand, it's unlikely that these diverse influences are all equal partners in embarrassment, and there are good reasons to wonder which of them, if any, is the most fundamental cause of the emotion. One reason is practicality. If we are to help people who are burdened by an excessive susceptibility to embarrassment, we need to know where to work. The dramaturgic model implies that social skill training may be an effective inoculation against embarrassment; presumably, the more deft and skilled one is, the less awkwardness one will feel during a given predicament and the more quickly normal interaction can be restored. In contrast, the social evaluation model suggests that people try to be less concerned with what others think of them, pointing to cognitive rather than behavioral interventions. Moreover, the self-esteem view suggests that we bolster self-esteem rather than defuse others' evaluations, and the personal standards model implies that self-esteem is immaterial as long as our ideals become less strict. Obviously, it would be a waste of time and money to address all of these issues if only one of them is key.

Just as compelling for us scientists, however, is the theoretical ambiguity itself. Our ability to assess meaningfully the empirical fitness of these four perspectives speaks to the essential quality of our knowledge. We truly understand embarrassment only when we can pinpoint its causes. Thus it is worthwhile to compare and contrast these models of embarrassment more thoroughly to determine whether any one of them is more capable than the others.

## Personal Standards Revisited

The personal standards perspective probably faces more empirical peril than the other three models of embarrassment. People do typically feel inferior and incompetent when they are embarrassed (Parrott & Smith, 1991), but other aspects of ordinary embarrassment do not fit the standards model particularly well.

For one thing, people very rarely experience embarrassment when they are alone (Parrott & Smith, 1991; Tangney et al., 1996). If embarrassment were not tied to interpersonal, public events as the other three models suggest, it would undoubtedly occur more often as we commit various blunders when others are absent. To the contrary, however, many events that do embarrass us would not cause the same reaction if no one else were aware of them, suggesting that more than private standards are at stake.

Here's an example: I have a steep driveway at my home that meets the street at a bad angle, and if I'm not careful as I leave in the morning, I'm likely to spill coffee from my customary travel mug onto my clothes. I've tried it both ways, and I assure you that sloshing hot coffee into my lap is embarrassing if someone else is present, but only annoying and frustrating when I'm alone. In fact, I'm never embarrassed by my clumsy behavior unless it is witnessed by or will later become known to others.[1]

On occasion, people do report being embarrassed when no one else is present (Tangney et al., 1996). However, as we argued earlier (in Chapter 3), such events inevitably involve either the prospect of discovery by others or the invention of an imaginary, disapproving audience. They may be objectively private events, but their emotional consequences appear to result from vividly anticipating others' reactions. Close inspection of hundreds and hundreds of embarrassments (Stonehouse & Miller, 1994) finds no examples of the kind of solitary embarrassment that the personal standards model suggests should be fairly common.

It's true that people *can* be embarrassed when they violate personal standards for their behavior that others do not share. If you reexamine this category of embarrassment (i.e., Departures from Personal Goals) in Chapter 4, however, you'll find that people always believed they were in public predicaments, even if they were not, when they experienced such embarrassments. In such cases, individuals had not met their own stringent criteria for social grace, weight loss, or tidiness. In our judgment (Stonehouse & Miller, 1994), they really hadn't broken any consensual social norms, but they thought they had and *they assumed that these transgressions were obvious to their audiences*. It did not appear that such embarrassments were based in private distress over their failed ideals at all.

In fact, no study has been able to demonstrate that violations of personal standards have any effect on embarrassment that does not involve the influences proposed by the other models. Indeed, the few investigations that have specifically explored the personal standards approach have found it difficult to create situations that violate standards but that do not also involve awkward interactions or threatening social evaluations. For instance, Babcock and Sabini (1990, p. 161) used scenarios such as the following to violate the standards of their subjects:

> [Imagine that] you've been flirting on the phone with someone you are really interested in. . . . As soon as you hang up, the phone rings again. You are sure that it must be your "sweetheart" again. You say in a sexy voice, "I knew that you wouldn't be able to stand being without me for long." You expect to hear a sexy reply back. You get a reply and you recognize the voice, but it's your mother's.

People found this event embarrassing, but it obviously presented both interactive and evaluative dilemmas—What to say next? Oh no, what is Mom thinking?—in addition to portraying a personal mistake, so the source of any resultant embarrassment was unclear. All the examples of standards violations Babcock and Sabini were able to devise allowed similar ambiguities.

Worse, it seems to me that the embarrassing potential of an event like this actually supports other models of embarrassment better than the standards model. Imagine making the same mistake in judgment in the phone scenario but having the second caller turn out to be a close friend with whom you've shared sexy secrets and who knows of your attraction to your "sweetheart." The identical personal error, the same private malfeasance, would be much less embarrassing and would probably trigger an excited discussion of what went on in the prior phone call. However, if the severity of embarrassment that results from a behavior depends on the nature of the audience that witnesses it (as of course it does; see Chapter 3), interpersonal influences beyond one's own personal standards for conduct must be involved.

Our surveys of embarrassing predicaments (Miller, 1992; Stonehouse & Miller, 1994) pointed to other problems in applying the personal standards model, which seemed to fit some embarrassments poorly. For instance, what personal violations are at work when someone really hasn't misbehaved at all and embarrassment results from audience provocation? People can be embarrassed by unwarranted teasing that they do not deserve, and such predicaments seem to involve personal standards only obliquely, if at all.

At bottom, then, no data provide particular support for the personal standards model, and there are aspects of embarrassment that are inconsistent with it. The model's adherents may be correct in arguing that people don't like to deviate from the "guidelines" that specify how they "should act in a given situation" (Babcock & Sabini, 1990, p. 154), but it may be more useful to conceive of these guidelines as the impressions people wish to make on others—and thus as *interpersonal* standards that vary from audience to audience—than as private, personal standards that are consistent across situations. Each of the other three models of embarrassment makes this assumption, and each of them does a better job of explaining embarrassment.

## Situational Self-Esteem Reconsidered

Like the personal standards perspective, Modigliani's (1971) situational self-esteem model holds that our personal judgments of our behavior play a fundamental role in producing embarrassment. Unlike the standards approach, however, the self-esteem view suggests that we temporarily come to view ourselves negatively because of our concern over what others may be thinking of us. An audience's unwanted evaluations are thought to cause the momentary reduction in self-esteem that in turn causes embarrassment, and, with this view, the self-esteem model does a better job than the standards model of accounting for the predominately public nature of embarrassment. Moreover, as we have seen, people do tend to feel negatively about themselves, feeling inept and incompetent, when they are embarrassed (Parrott & Smith, 1991). Nevertheless, the self-esteem view may be a bit off the mark: Studies that have pitted self-evaluations against audience evaluations (or self-esteem versus "social-esteem") as predictors of embarrassment consistently find that embarrassment is more closely related to what we think others think of us than to what we think of ourselves.

In one early study, British researchers Tony Manstead and Gün Semin (1981) found that college students who imagined themselves in various embarrassing predicaments—including one dear to my heart (see Chapter 1), spilling a drink over some strangers in a pub—did not judge their own behavior as negatively as they believed others did. The students consistently believed that observers would judge them more harshly than they were judging themselves. Public transgressions thus seemed to do more damage to a person's social image, or "face," than to the person's self-esteem.

Jerry Parrott and Stefanie Smith (1991) obtained similar results when they collected accounts of actual embarrassment along with reports of situational self-esteem and social evaluation from 60 young adults. Parrott and Smith asked their respondents to provide detailed descriptions of a past embarrassment along with formal ratings of what they were feeling at the time. Some of these ratings assessed self-esteem (e.g., "I thought poorly of myself in this situation") and others tapped concern with others' opinions (e.g., "I was worried about how others would evaluate me"). In general, the remembered embarrassments were characterized more by perceived drops in social-esteem than by any change in self-esteem. Instead of dwelling on self-rebuke and criticism, people typically worried more about what others were thinking during an embarrassing episode.

These results do not preclude the possibility that negative social evaluations have their effects by influencing self-esteem as Modigliani (1971) suggested, but they do argue that embarrassed people are more concerned with their social images than with their self-esteem. It also appears that substantial harm to a person's social image may not always produce corresponding damage to that person's self-esteem. This is how Manstead and Semin (1981, p. 255) interpreted their results, asserting that "the actor experiences tension, embarrassment, anxiety, etc., because he or she imagines that others evaluate him/her more negatively as a consequence of the witnessed blunder, despite the fact that the actor's self-image is unaffected by the incident."

Still, the relative influences of self-evaluation and social evaluation in producing embarrassment were somewhat uncertain, so I tried to clarify the issue with an experiment that manipulated both variables (Miller, 1996). I asked 143 college students to imagine that they had to give a speech to a class just as they were coming down with the flu. They felt woozy and rotten, and their professor was sympathetic, but there was no way to reschedule the talk. Some of the students then envisioned the talk going badly, with a long, awkward pause at one point when they lost their train of thought; when they finished, they felt they had done a poor job. Others imagined the talk going surprisingly well, with a long, poised pause for dramatic effect, and they returned to their seats thinking they had done a fine job. Regardless of their own evaluations of their performances, however, one of three social evaluations awaited them once they sat down. A third of the participants were asked to picture a classmate leaning over and criticizing them, saying, "Hey, didn't you have time to prepare for your talk? We all thought you'd do better than that." Other students visualized an unwanted evaluation that was softened by sympathy: "It was a shame you had to give your talk today; we could see you weren't feeling well." Finally, the remaining students envisioned unabashed praise: "Hey, that was a really nice talk. I especially liked the dramatic pause." The procedure of the study thus compared and contrasted a favorable or unfavorable *self*-evaluation of a public performance with a positive, negative, or sympathetically negative *social* evaluation of the same performance.

The students described how they thought they would feel in such situations, and the self-evaluations they envisioned had two important effects. First, a self-esteem scale showed that their self-evaluations did influence their situational self-esteem; in particular, the negative self-evaluation students felt that they had done poorly in that situation. Second, as Modigliani (1971) would expect, the students with the lower situational self-esteem did expect to be more embarrassed by their performances than their prouder counterparts were. The students' own judgments of their public behavior did affect their level of embarrassment independently of what others were thinking.

However, the social evaluations from the audience had a much *larger* effect on the students' embarrassment. Even if they privately felt they had done a fine job, the students expected to be quite embarrassed by learning that others thought them inept. These data did not seem to fit the situational self-esteem model especially well. The three audience reactions—the positive judgment, the sympathetic negative judgment, and the negative evaluation—each caused a different (and successively higher) level of embarrassment, and they had an influence that was 12 times larger than that of situational self-esteem. Moreover, the social evaluations did not directly affect the students' self-esteem, as Modigliani expected that they should.

I think the results argue that our self-evaluations can play a role in producing embarrassment, but that the chain of events is not what Modigliani proposed. Low situational self-esteem does not appear to be the primary cause of embarrassment as Modigliani suggested. Instead, it seems to play a secondary role, perhaps influencing embarrassment by increasing the threats presented by its more central causes (such as awkward interaction or unwanted social evaluations) without being an essential ingredient itself. For instance, my analysis of embarrassability (Miller, 1995b) did show that people with chronically low self-esteem were more embarrassable than those who regarded themselves more highly. However, susceptibility to embarrassment depended more on persistent concern about what others were thinking than on what one thought of oneself. People with low self-esteem also tended to have higher fears of negative social evaluation, and dispositional self-esteem per se did not predict a person's embarrassability once the person's fear of negative evaluation was taken into account. Indeed, even people with high self-esteem were quite embarrassable if they worried too much about others' evaluations.

Similarly, in my experiment (Miller, 1996), people who felt good about their performances became embarrassed if they learned that others disapproved, and social evaluations were much more influential than self-evaluations. It appears that, regardless of what *we're* thinking of our actions, the realization that others have judged us ill can be instantly abashing.

The key point here is that negative self-evaluations may intensify embarrassment, but they are not necessary for it to occur. Although we may often feel badly about ourselves during embarrassing predicaments, embarrassment can occur even though we are privately sure of ourselves. The empirical studies that bear on this point support Charles Darwin's assertion penned more than a century ago: "It is not the simple act of reflecting on our own appearance, but the thinking what others think of us, which excites a blush" (1873/1965, p. 325).

## The Real Contenders

Private, personal standards do not seem to be much involved in embarrassment, and situational self-esteem, while somewhat influential, plays a tangential role. That leaves two explanations for embarrassment that spring directly from Goffman's (1959) analysis of social life, with both assuming that embarrassment hinges on the presence of others, either as interactive partners or as evaluative critics. In fact, together, the dramaturgic model and the social evaluation model speak to the two most central features of prototypical embarrassment. When Parrott and Smith (1991) asked 61 young adults to describe a "typical" embarrassment, (1) flustered, awkward indecision and (2) dread of what others were thinking were the two components of the emotion most likely to be mentioned.

Because they revolve around these central ingredients, both the dramaturgic and the evaluation models are consistent with most of what we know about embarrassment. Both are useful perspectives. Nevertheless, I think it has become clear that one is a richer, more complete explanation of embarrassment than the other. One of them comes closer to identifying the fundamental cause of embarrassment. Let's see which is the better.

*Dramaturgy Reexamined*

Embarrassment *feels* awkward, of course, and there's no question that awkward interactions can cause people to feel embarrassed. We found such instances in our surveys of embarrassing predicaments (see Chapter 4), and Jerry Parrott, John Sabini, and Maury Silver (1988) have demonstrated the embarrassing potential of awkward interactions in an ingenious experiment. Parrott and his colleagues asked college students to imagine that they were being refused a date for one of three different reasons. In one scenario, they envisioned being told that their potential date was already involved with someone else and was refusing any other offers. This was a reasonable explanation that was not particularly demeaning, and it was not expected to be very embarrassing. In contrast, in another condition, the students imagined their invitations being bluntly rebuffed with a terse refusal. This obvious rejection was expected to be embarrassing because it both created an awkward interaction and endangered the recipient's social esteem. However, in a third, key condition, the students envisioned being refused with an ostensibly legitimate, publicly acceptable reason that they privately knew to be a lie: The potential date said that he or she was already involved with someone else, but the student knew that that was not true. This was a "transparent pretext" for refusing the date. It was an innocuous explanation but it was blatantly false, and Parrott et al. believed that it would create a threat to social esteem without disrupting the encounter and creating an awkward interaction; the pretext would presumably allow the interaction to continue as if nothing bad had happened, even though the students would privately know they had been rejected. Parrott et al.

thus suggested that the dramaturgic model would not predict much embarrassment in the transparent pretext condition whereas the social evaluation model would.

The students' reports of the embarrassment they would feel in each of these situations demonstrated that, indeed, the refusal disguised by the transparent pretext caused less embarrassment than the outright snub. A clear-cut rebuff was more embarrassing than a pretense that was less disruptive, even though both situations posed a threat to social esteem. Parrott and his colleagues (1988) argued that this is just what the dramaturgic model would predict, and asserted that the results tied embarrassment more closely to dramaturgic concerns than to worries about social evaluation. Combined with the obvious feelings of discombobulation and clumsiness that characterize embarrassment (Parrott & Smith, 1991), these data led Parrott et al. to conclude that embarrassment results more from anxious uncertainty and a loss of direction in social interaction than it does from concerns over what others are thinking of us.

### Social Evaluation Strikes Back

I wasn't so sure. Parrott et al.'s (1988) results would be troublesome for a social evaluation perspective if the transparent pretext and the curt rebuff created similar threats to a person's social image but caused different levels of embarrassment. However, it seemed to me that the pretext was a kinder method of refusal that communicated higher regard for the recipient than the blunt refusal did, and thus posed a weaker threat to one's social esteem. If that were so, the social evaluation model would also predict the results Parrott et al. obtained.

I didn't think that the data conclusively linked embarrassment to dramaturgic woes. I was impressed with Parrott et al.'s procedure, however, and used an adaptation of it in my own attempt to disentangle the overlapping predictions of the two theoretical models (Miller, 1996). Like Parrott et al., I asked college students to imagine being refused a date for an innocuous, benign reason, or for a kindly but transparently false reason that was more threatening. In my procedure, however, they further imagined that the news of the refusal was conveyed to them by a messenger who also obviously believed the refusal to be threatening or benign. The students' own perceptions of the situation were independent of those of the messenger, so four different scenarios were possible.

In one combination, which was likely to arouse both dramaturgic and social evaluative concerns, the students learned that they had been spurned through an uncomfortable interaction with a messenger who also knew of their rejection. In contrast, in another case, the students knew they had been rebuffed but learned of their rejection in an innocent interchange with a messenger who accepted the pretext for the refusal and saw nothing wrong. This situation was likely to involve an unwanted evaluation in the context of an interaction that was not particularly awkward at all. In a third combination, the messenger thought the students had been snubbed, but the students themselves saw nothing amiss, creating an awkward interaction without a negative evaluation from the person who refused the date. Finally, in a fourth situation, neither the students nor the messenger perceived the refusal to be threatening, believing that the date was turned down simply because the other person had a class to attend.

The procedure thus manipulated the apparent favorability of a salient social evaluation (from the person refusing the date) independently of the awkwardness of the current interaction. Thereafter, once they had contemplated these events, the students told me how embarrassed they thought they would be in each of them. The results supported the assumptions of the dramaturgic model; a difficult interaction with a messenger who thought (correctly or not) that the students had been snubbed was more embarrassing than an interaction that was more mundane. However, a threatening rejection was even more embarrassing, whether or not that rejection was apparent to the current interactive partner. The sudden recognition of an unwanted social evaluation was embarrassing whether or not it was accompanied by a maladroit interaction and its potential loss of script.

Social evaluation processes can evidently create embarrassment in the absence of dramaturgic difficulty. On the other hand, it may be harder for a dramaturgic dilemma to cause embarrassment without simultaneously creating unwanted evaluations. You may have already realized that the same manipulation that made the interaction with the messenger more or less awkward in my procedure (by varying what the messenger was said to think about the refusal) may also have influenced the messenger's presumed evaluation of the student getting the news. Thus, awkwardness did affect embarrassment but it may have done so, in part, by changing the evaluative climate of the interaction in which it occurred. My procedure demonstrated that unwanted evaluation can produce embarrassment independently of awkwardness, but it's not clear that awkwardness can create embarrassment independently of unwanted evaluation.

In any case, in my study, concern over social evaluation was a more potent cause of embarrassment than awkward uncertainty was; the social evaluation manipulation explained twice as much variance in the students' expected embarrassment as the dramaturgic variable did (Miller, 1996). This result, coupled with the real possibility that awkward interactions are embarrassing mostly because they make bad impressions on others, led me to conclude that concerns over social evaluation are the more fundamental source of embarrassment.

This is not to say that the flustered uncertainty that can result when interactions go awry is unimportant. Erving Goffman noted that a lack of poise is a very real threat to desirable interaction: "Face-to-face interaction in *any* culture seems to require just those capacities that flustering seems guaranteed to destroy. . . . Flustering threatens the encounter itself by disrupting the smooth transmission and reception by which encounters are sustained" (1956, p. 266). Because it is so disruptive, an awkward loss of script may be intrinsically aversive, just as Parrott et al. (1988) suggested. Moreover, as we have noted, such interruptions can also convey unwanted impressions. Goffman himself asserted that "to appear flustered, in our society at least, is considered evidence of weakness, inferiority, low status, moral guilt, defeat, and other unenviable attributes" (1956, p. 266). Thus, a sudden loss of script that leaves one at sea may quickly create concerns about what others may be thinking. On the other hand, a sudden concern over unwanted social evaluation can rob one of poise and grace and make one more awkward. In this way, the influences posited by the dramaturgic and social evaluation models probably interact and exacerbate each other in actual public predicaments, with each helping to make embarrassment worse.

Still, when the two influences are compared nose to nose, social evaluation is a more potent cause of embarrassment than awkward uncertainty is. Goffman believed this, I think, stating that "whatever else, embarrassment has to do with the figure the individual cuts before others felt to be there at the time. The crucial concern is the impression one makes on others in the present" (1956, pp. 264–265). For Goffman, the images we present to others were a fundamental concern in social life, and, as he suggested, embarrassment seems to spring, elementally, from our apprehension of what others are thinking of us. My study (Miller, 1996) suggests this conclusion, but there are several other findings that make the same point.

## A Broader View

In fact, I believe that our collected knowledge of embarrassment fits the social evaluation perspective better than any other model. Let me remind you of some of the things we've learned about embarrassment thus far.

*Embarrassing Circumstances.* Any of the four theoretical models needs to be stretched a bit to encompass all of the diverse events that can cause embarrassment, but the social evaluation model seems more elastic than the other perspectives. For instance, consider the example with which we started Chapter 1. "Marie" was embarrassed when she lost control of her slip and found it tangled around her ankles while she was crossing a busy intersection. For a moment she may have been at a loss for what to do in that situation, but I don't think that an aversive loss of script explains the embarrassment that washed over her. She would have faced the same instant of indecision over what to do if the street had been fogbound and her behavior had been invisible. Without witnesses, however, the failure of her slip would not have been very embarrassing. Instead, it is far more likely that she became embarrassed because of her acute dread over the image she was presenting to the anonymous witnesses watching her from their cars. She was in no sort of organized interaction that came wrenching to a halt, and she wasn't even sure that anyone else had noticed her predicament; nevertheless, the sudden threat of unwanted evaluation, even from unseen strangers, was enough to produce embarrassment.

Various situations that cause embarrassment are like this, involving undesired social evaluations from distant observers. Events such as a stumble on an icy sidewalk seen by someone a block away, or a child's mistake in the school play that embarrasses the parent watching from the wings, impose few dramaturgic consequences on an embarrassed person who is yards away from anyone else. The dramaturgic model hardly seems to apply. I suppose a proponent of the dramaturgic perspective could argue that people still experience aversive arousal in such situations because of their uncertainty about how to react, but that proposition begs the question of why people are so motivated to maintain a poised image for distant strangers. In such cases, even the dramaturgic model has to rely on the parsimonious answer provided by the social evaluation perspective: People care what others are thinking of them. Given that that is true, it seems unnecessary to include the additional assumptions required by the dramaturgic model to explain the embarrassing potential of such events. Whether or not they disrupt an ongoing public "performance," events like these create the potential for disapproval from others and are probably embarrassing because we care what others are thinking and dread unwanted evaluations so much.

Indeed, because embarrassing circumstances usually portray people in some undesired way, the social evaluation model provides a straightforward foundation for almost all of the events people find embarrassing. Even cases such as conspicuousness and overpraise—in which unwanted evaluations do not clearly result—can be explained with little effort if we assume that situations consistently associated with embarrassment can gradually become embarrassing themselves. As we saw in Chapter

5, Arnold Buss (1980) has argued that children slowly come to dread occasions in which they are the conspicuous objects of others' attention because such occasions so often result in ridicule and censure. Over time, as they become increasingly familiar with such situations, people may experience embarrassment when they "stick out like a sore thumb" even before any obvious disapproval results. In this fashion, embarrassment may occur even when one is being complimented and applauded if one is made conspicuous by the acclaim. (Presumably, if we consistently received lots of praise, we could learn that such conspicuousness is usually rewarding, and honors and tributes would slowly lose their power to embarrass us. Unfortunately, I doubt that many of us will get the chance to find out if that's true!)

Unwanted evaluations are also absent in instances of empathic embarrassment that occur when a person merely witnesses someone else's embarrassing predicament. However, empathic embarrassment depends on the observer's ability to imagine what the embarrassed target is feeling; it tends not to occur if the observer adopts a detached, dispassionate mindset (Miller, 1987). In fact, the surest way to induce empathic embarrassment is to get someone thinking, "Gosh, what would I be feeling if that were happening to me?" Innocent bystanders may not really be at risk of unwanted social evaluations when empathic embarrassment occurs, but a little imagination and their own potent experiences with social disapproval can remind them of how it feels. The fascinating result, which speaks to the power of embarrassment in social life, is that people can be vicariously unsettled simply by watching embarrassing circumstances befall someone else.

In sum, then, any theoretical model needs an impressive reach to encompass all of the various events that cause embarrassment. The social evaluation model provides that range, however, and is a more compact perspective that pertains more readily to more embarrassing circumstances than the dramaturgic model does. I think it fits other data better, as well.

*The Audience's Knowledge.* When we discuss how people respond to embarrassing predicaments in Chapter 9, we'll find that embarrassment can affect subsequent behavior outside the situations in which it occurs. Robert Apsler (1975) found that, once they had been embarrassed, research participants went to some trouble to make good impressions on people who didn't even know of their prior predicament. Embarrassment seemed to create a motive for desired evaluations that had carryover effects on entirely new interactions in which nothing was going wrong. The social evaluation model can readily account for this finding, but it's a little harder for the dramaturgic model to explain. From a dramaturgic perspective, once a wholly new, stable interaction with a new audience begins, recent embarrassments should be forgotten, but they're not.

*Developmental Processes.* As we've seen, the capacity for embarrassment unfolds over time, and youngsters may not experience "mature" embarrassment until they are nearly 11 years old (Bennett, 1989). The dramaturgic model would suggest that embarrassment develops gradually because it takes time to learn the rules of interaction and to establish reliable expectations for social intercourse. Presumably it is only when those expectations and scripts have been thoroughly learned and rehearsed that violations of those scripts cause full-fledged embarrassment.

However, I think the social evaluation perspective provides more elegant explanations for two developmental facts. First, the initial, primordial signs of embarrassment correspond closely to the emergence of public self-consciousness (Lewis, 1995), which should occur, according to the social evaluation model, as children first become aware of themselves as social objects. In contrast, from a dramaturgic perspective, it's nothing more than a coincidence of maturation that public self-consciousness and embarrassment are linked. Second, a social evaluation view holds that embarrassment takes a decade to emerge in mature form because fully envisioning others' judgments of oneself is a complex cognitive feat that requires an advanced stage of perspective taking and cognitive development. Learning the rules of interaction seems a simpler talent, and a dramaturgic model should expect mature embarrassment to emerge sooner than it does.

*Embarrassability.* We've also seen that susceptibility to embarrassment is associated with low skill at impression management; people who are more embarrassable are less deft at managing their interactions, just as the dramaturgic model suggests (Miller, 1995b). On the other hand, you learn far more about a person's embarrassability by examining the person's fear of negative evaluation and attentiveness to social norms than you do by measuring the person's interactive dexterity. In general, highly embarrassable people dread public violations of social norms and expect fearsome disapproval when such violations occur, a pattern that is clearly consistent with the social evaluation model of embarrassment.

The personality traits that regulate a person's responses to an embarrassing predicament may not necessarily be similar to the situational influences that cause the emotion in the first place. Nevertheless, although dramaturgic difficulty is influential, studies of embarrassability imply that concern over social evaluations is the more central component of embarrassment. As I argued elsewhere, "whatever their dramaturgic abilities, it appears that if people were heedless of others' opinions, they would not be very embarrassable" (Miller, 1995a, p. 326).

## The Nature of Embarrassment

Indeed, people generally agree that they are worried about what others are thinking of them when they become embarrassed. Parrott and Smith (1991) found that both dramaturgic distress (e.g., "I didn't know how to act") and social evaluative concern (e.g., "I was worried about how others would evaluate me") are characteristic of people's accounts of actual past embarrassments. However, Parrott and Smith also determined that concern over social evaluation is *more characteristic* of people's description of a "typical" episode of embarrassment than is dramaturgic uncertainty, a loss of situational self-esteem, or a violation of personal standards. It appears that people do feel awkward when they are embarrassed but that they do not believe that such awkwardness epitomizes the state. Instead, the most essential ingredient in people's prototypes of embarrassment is dread of what others are thinking.

This belief holds among embarrassment researchers, too; the social evaluation model of embarrassment is the favorite among social scientists (e.g., Edelmann, 1987; Leary & Kowalski, 1995; Scheff, 1990; Semin & Manstead, 1981). On the basis of this consensus and the data we have reviewed, I think it's reasonable to assert that embarrassing circumstances often leave us uncertain of what to say and do next, but that such uncertainty is not a necessary precursor of embarrassment. Rather, the more fundamental source of embarrassed emotion is our realization that unwanted events may have left others with undesired impressions of us, and, in most cases, it is this threat that causes both embarrassment and the dramaturgic distress that accompanies it.

Here, then, is the resolution of our theoretical quest: Embarrassment is *the acute state of flustered, awkward, abashed chagrin that follows events that increase the threat of unwanted evaluations from real or imagined audiences*. This perspective does not deny the possibility that dramaturgic distress, blows to situational self-esteem, and violations of personal standards can exacerbate embarrassment when they are present, but it does assert that they are not needed for embarrassment to occur. The only necessary condition for embarrassment is acute concern about social evaluation.

This assumption has been a theme of this book thus far, and it will be useful to us again in the three final chapters. For the moment, however, there's one last piece of unfinished business. We've seen that embarrassment is a pervasive emotion that occurs around the world, and I've now formally tied it to apprehension about what others may be thinking of us. What's still missing is an explanation of why people should be so affected by the judgments of others. Why is an openness to embarrassment a ubiquitous human condition?

## THE BIG PICTURE

Unwanted social evaluations may cause us emotional distress because they bear on a basic, universal human motivation, the *need to belong*. Theorists Roy Baumeister and Mark Leary (1995, p. 522) have argued that "human beings are fundamentally and pervasively motivated by a need to belong, that is, by a strong desire to form and maintain enduring interpersonal attachments." According to this view, our species is "naturally driven toward establishing and sustaining belongingness" (p. 499), and the desire to attain some minimum level of acceptance from, and closeness to, a sufficient number of others may be the prepotent interpersonal motive that guides our social behavior.

In defense of this claim, Baumeister and Leary showed that humans readily form relational bonds with others, spend considerable time thinking about their relationships, resist the dissolution of their existing attachments, and suffer various forms of physical and mental maladies if their belongingness needs are not met. For all of these reasons, the need to belong is intimately tied to our emotions, so that "even potential threats to social bonds generate a variety of unpleasant emotional states" (p. 520). Negative affect is common when people face any kind of real or imagined rejection from others.

Baumeister and Leary even speculated that the human need to belong is much more than a learned desire that emerges from our rewarding experiences with others; instead, it may be innate. Such a motive presumably became ingrained in our species because it was evolutionarily adaptive, conferring survival and reproductive benefits on our forebears who followed its constraints. In our dim ancestral past, when conditions were harsh and survival was uncertain, those humans who were cast out of their living and social groups may have been relatively unlikely to shape future generations by having children and passing on their genes. Those who were shunned and rejected by others may have had to fear for their lives. By contrast, those who sought appropriate attachments with others and met the standards for inclusion in their social groups would have been much more likely to survive and prosper.

Concern over acceptance from others may literally have been a matter of life and death. Significant departures from established norms may have been matters of grave consequence to be dreaded and feared.

As a result, our ancestors may have been anxious to avoid such blunders and to demonstrate their continuing competency and desirability to their fellows. In such environments it would have been useful and perhaps inevitable for people to gradually develop negative reactions to circumstances like those that cause embarrassment. Arousal and emotion may have become routine "whenever some event, or even some implication about the self, raises the threat of social rejection or interpersonal failure" (Baumeister & Tice, 1990, p. 183). Moreover, it would have been advantageous, both to avoid such negative emotions and to maximize one's long-term prospects for survival, to "learn and conform to the standards, rules, and norms of their culture because these embody the criteria for inclusion and exclusion" (Baumeister & Tice, 1990, p. 183). Of course, it is precisely the violations of these standards and rules that cause embarrassment.

Thus I think it is reasonable to think of embarrassment as one manifestation of the fundamental human need to seek inclusion and to avoid rejection in our dealings with our fellows. The concern over social evaluation from which embarrassment springs is a plausible result of this need, and it makes sense that an emotion such as embarrassment should follow the unwanted evaluations that pose the threat of worrisome rejection (Leary, 1990). By making people sensitive to the opinions of their fellows, embarrassment may have helped alert people to any criticism that forewarned abandonment. Over the eons, embarrassment may have become the useful "social counterpart to physical pain; just as it would be hard to survive if we had no pain to warn us of threats to our physical well-being, we would not last long if we had no social anxiety or embarrassment to warn us of possible rebuke and rejection" (Miller & Leary, 1992, p. 216).

Leary and his colleagues have also argued that even our own self-esteem, our chronic positive or negative evaluation of ourselves, reflects the status of our acceptance by others (Leary & Downs, 1995; Leary, Schreindorfer, & Haupt, 1995; Leary, Tambor, Terdal, & Downs, 1995). Events that damage self-esteem also result in rejection by others, and interpersonal rejections cause decreases in self-esteem that do not result when the rejection is impersonal or random. For Leary, self-esteem is much like a social evaluative fuel gauge; it is high when we are confident that *others* hold us in high regard, but low when we fear that others are unimpressed. A predominant human need for belongingness presumably requires some systematic means of monitoring others' reactions to oneself, and Leary suggested that self-esteem serves that very function.

These bold ideas all suggest that awareness of what others may be thinking of us is never far from our minds. We may be absorbed by other things, of course, and may often—though temporarily—give no heed to others' evaluations of us. Still, our immediate, involuntary responses to situations that increase the salience of social evaluation suggest that our species is especially attentive to the judgments of our conspecifics. Indeed, back in 1922, sociologist Charles Cooley asserted that a concern over social evaluation was

> in one form or another, the mainspring of endeavor and a chief interest of the imagination throughout life. As is the case with other feelings, we do not think much of it so long as it is moderately and regularly gratified. Many people of balanced mind and congenial activity scarcely know that they care what others think of them and will deny, perhaps with indignation, that such care is an important factor in what they are and do. But this is illusion. If failure or disgrace arrives, if one suddenly finds that the faces of men show coldness or contempt instead of the kindliness and deference that he is used to, he will perceive from the shock, the fear, the sense of being outcast and helpless, that he was living in the minds of others without knowing it, just as we daily walk the solid ground without thinking how it bears us up. (1922/1964, p. 208)

There are other, less grand, reasons why the failures of impression management that cause embarrassment may be disconcerting (Geen, 1991). For one thing, by successfully making desired impressions on others we often gain some control over how we are treated by them. Unwanted lapses in impression management may be straightforwardly punishing when they result in the loss of anticipated social or material gains. Furthermore, because our self-presentations are often heartfelt attempts to communicate our personal conceptions of ourselves to others (Leary, 1995), it can be particularly demeaning to have others scoff at what they see. These occasional influences can be subsumed by the broad, innate drive to avoid rejection from others that is postulated by the need to belong, however, and the dread of social evaluation that characterizes embarrassment seems to be more consistent with that larger human need.

Thus our capacity for embarrassment may exemplify our humanity. It is possible that embarrassment shares an ancient evolutionary origin with a fundamental human need that has come to epitomize our species. Several other animals live solitary lives, joining their fellows only now and then to reproduce, but humans are more gregarious creatures who strive to maintain some minimal level of social acceptance and inclusion. They are sensitive to rejection and potential exclusion, and thus are susceptible to the embarrassment that follows the threat of unwanted social evaluations.

This is not a bad thing, however. Remarkably, embarrassment seems to be much more than a mere demonstration of our chagrin at unwanted predicaments; as a public, social emotion, it also provides a means of managing and repairing those predicaments. Embarrassment not only results from our human need to belong, it provides an emergency means of helping to fulfill it, as we'll see in the next two chapters.

## CHAPTER 8

# Signs of Embarrassment

One of the most remarkable features of embarrassment is that it is such a public event. Most of our embarrassments are apparent to others. We lose our calm composure when embarrassment strikes; even the most stoic people may avert their eyes, shift uncomfortably, and blush involuntarily. As a result, an episode of embarrassment may be plainly evident to total strangers. If an audience is close at hand, our sheepish chagrin at some transgression may be unmistakable. Moreover, we may have very little control over our public displays of abashed behavior so that, even if we desperately wish to appear unruffled, our embarrassment may be obvious.

Indeed, embarrassment's public nature gives it a character that is quite distinct from some other emotions that are private experiences that can occur when one is totally alone. Embarrassment is a social, *interpersonal* event that depends on the presence of others. Accordingly, it may be useful to think of embarrassment not only as a painful personal response to untoward public events but as a vivid interpersonal *communication* that also informs others of our dismay and chagrin. The emotion itself may exist not only to alert us to the threat of unwanted evaluations, but to provide a reliable public signal of our distress as well.

This provocative notion has emerged from studies of the interactive consequences of embarrassment. As we'll see, embarrassment usually changes the situations in which it occurs, often having substantial impact on what people do and say next. It has such effects, in part, because bystanders are so likely to be aware of a person's embarrassment when it occurs. There are a variety of expressive signals that may reliably inform bystanders that someone is embarrassed, and foremost among them is the most dramatic, most peculiar, and most uncontrollable of them all: the blush.

## BLUSHING

Blushing has been of interest to scientists for generations. Charles Darwin (1872/1965) believed blushing to be "the most human of all expressions" (p. 309) and "common to most, probably to all, of the races of man" (p. 320). (He obviously agreed with his contemporary, Mark Twain [1897, p. 238], who wryly observed that "Man is the Only Animal that Blushes. Or needs to.") Because he knew that even blind people blush, Darwin maintained that people were born with a capacity for blushing. On the other hand, he also knew that young infants do not blush, and, impressively, he tied blushing to the emergence of public self-consciousness, and a person's ultimate dread of others' appraisals, more than 120 years before researchers began formally investigating the social evaluation model of embarrassment.

However, Darwin had difficulty explaining why blushing only occurs in the upper chest, neck, and face. Admitting some uncertainty, he suggested that blushing was limited to those locations because the threat of unwanted social evaluations led people to focus their attention on the specific parts of their bodies—their faces—that were ordinarily visible to others. This focused attention, in turn, supposedly influenced the "tonic contractions" of one's capillaries, causing more blood to flow to those parts of the body. Of course, this early view was a bit naive; there is no modern evidence that merely thinking hard about part of one's body encourages more blood to rush there.[1]

Other explanations for blushing have assumed that blood flow to the face increases for different reasons. The Freudian psychodynamic tradition has produced a variety of proposals, all generally holding that blushing is the visible manifestation of unfulfilled impulses and/or repressed intrapsychic conflicts (see Karch, 1971). One such suggestion was that blushing occurred when sexual arousal was displaced away from the genitals and onto the face due to a fear of castration (Feldman, 1941). Another point of view held that blushing was the unwanted result of repressed urges toward exhibitionism; people who could not face (so to speak) their impulses to expose themselves to others displaced those desires into another noticeable form of public display, an obvious blush (Alexander, 1930). Of course, according to clinical psychologist and embarrassment expert Robert Edelmann (1987), only in "one's wildest imaginings" (p. 10) are these "fanciful" (p. 9) suppositions to be considered useful explanations of blushing. They have little to say about the interpersonal situations that really do cause blushing, and probably tell us more about the world view of psychodynamic theorists than they do about blushing itself.

In contrast, more modern analyses of blushing clearly acknowledge its social nature. In fact, a distinction is now commonly made between facial flushing, which can occur from impersonal events such as exercise, alcohol consumption, or menopausal "hot flashes," and blushing, which is "a spontaneous reddening or darkening of the face, ears, neck, and upper chest that occurs in response to perceived social scrutiny or evaluation" (Leary, Britt, Cutlip, & Templeton, 1992, p. 446). This remarkable reddening results from the dilation of the small blood vessels in the face that increases the volume of blood in the surface of the skin. That this singular reaction occurs at all is interesting, and that it so often accompanies embarrassment is fascinating.

However, Leary and his colleagues (1992) cautioned their readers against assuming that blushing and embarrassment always go hand in hand. They noted that blushing is always a social, public event but argued that it simply occurs when we encounter undue and undesired attention from others, whether or not that attention is embarrassing. For Leary, close inspection and observation of our current behavior by others is inherently threatening, arousing social evaluative concerns and self-awareness that can elicit blushing even when our behavior is impeccable. Leary et al. noted that simply accusing a person of blushing is often enough to stimulate a real blush, for instance, and blushes often occur when no obvious damage to a person's social identity has been done.

On the other hand, situations that involve undesired social attention invariably make the possibility of unwanted impressions more salient. As we've seen, several situations—such as those involving conspicuousness or overpraise—can be embarrassing even when one's behavior is not demonstrably deficient, presumably because similar close inspections of our behavior have so often been embarrassing in the past (see A. H. Buss, 1980, and Chapter 4). Undesired social attention is a necessary ingredient in embarrassing predicaments, and is itself a sufficient cause of some embarrassments, so I don't think the distinction between embarrassed and nonembarrassed blushing is quite as clear as Leary et al. (1992) suggested. Accusing people of unwarranted blushing as Leary has, for instance, is to charge them with an undesirable loss of control, creating a predicament where there was none. (As Leary et al. acknowledged, "blushing is damaging to one's image even if one has committed no obvious infraction" [p. 448].) I agree that people sometimes blush before a clearly unwanted impression is made on others, but I think it's very rare for blushing to occur in situations in which people are not aware of the potential for embarrassment. Furthermore, blushing and embarrassment share similar origins in concerns about what others are thinking of us, and blushing is reliable enough a sign of embarrassment that observers can justifiably assume that someone who is blushing is also (or is about to be) embarrassed.

Thus, blushing and embarrassment are not synonymous—each may occur without the other—but they overlap considerably. In particular, blushing rarely occurs in situations that do not trigger simultaneous embarrassment. On the whole, blushing is a reliable signal of embarrassment, a fact that raises several questions.

## How Do People Blush?

The precise physiological mechanisms underlying blushing are better understood now than in Darwin's day, but there are still points of ambiguity. Blushing may be visible in, and limited to, the face and neck for several interrelated reasons (Cutlip & Leary, 1993). First, the face contains an unusually high number of blood vessels near the surface of the skin. In addition, the face's vessels may be capable of carrying more blood than others of their size elsewhere in the body (Wilkin, 1988). These two features allow a sizable volume of blood to flow near the skin of the face when blushing occurs, causing a change in the color of the cheeks that may be apparent to others. In addition, the veins in the face are biologically prepared to accommodate such blood flow; they are rather atypical in containing neurochemical receptors controlling vaso-dilation that are not commonly found in veinous tissue (Mellander, Andersson, Afzelius, & Hellstrand, 1982).[2] These receptors can cause the vessels in the face to dilate and carry more blood during periods of moderate sympathetic nervous system arousal that cause other periph-eral vessels to constrict (Drummond, 1989). Thus when a person is aroused by unwanted social evaluation, his or her fingers may grow cooler (from reduced blood flow) even as a greater volume of blood warms the cheeks, causing a sensation of facial warmth that is often the person's only clue that he or she is blushing (Leary, Rejeski, et al., 1994; Shearn, Bergman, Hill, Abel, & Hinds, 1990, 1992). All of this happens automatically; blushing is an involuntary response that is beyond con-scious control. Indeed, people often blush noticeably without knowing that they are blushing at all (Leary et al., 1992).

If people do realize that they are blushing, other processes may come into play. First, because they fear that their blushing is making them more conspicuous, people can be embarrassed by their blushing as well as by the event that originally caused the blush; as a result, being even more embarrassed, they may blush even harder (Asendorpf, 1990; Edelmann, 1990a). Jens Asendorpf (1984) coined the term "secondary embarrassment" to describe this sort of vicious cycle, noting that people can sometimes be embarrassed about being embarrassed. A wry, fictional example of this was dreamed up by Jerry Scott (1989, p. B6), the creator of the comic strip "Nancy." In one strip, Nancy becomes embarrassed when her stomach gurgles loudly in class, and then realizes, "Oh no! My face is turning red and everyone is laughing! Now I'm embarrassed for being embarrassed!" Her problem continues: "Oh no! I can't stop turning red! I think I'm embarrassed about being embarrassed for being embarrassed!" The punchline, as she sinks in her chair, is "I wonder if the Guinness Book of World Records has a category for this. . . ." (They don't, but we do: It's a "loss of control.") In real life, such events are rarely humorous for the blusher, who often feels considerable chagrin at his or her conspicuous coloring (Edelmann, 1990a; Edelmann & Skov, 1993).

   In addition, in a more subtle mechanism, there may be visceral cues attached to blushing that exacerbate embarrassment. According to an intriguing *facial feedback* hypothesis, facial expressions both reflect emotional experiences and help to shape them. The idea is that, due to the intimate, innate connections between the brain and the musculature and vasculature of the face, certain facial responses may gradually cause real physiological changes in the brain that affect subsequent emotional experience. There is evidence, for instance, that pulling back the corners of one's mouth—simulating the muscle movements involved in smiling—by holding a pen between one's teeth (Strack, Martin, & Stepper, 1988) or pronouncing the letter "e" (Zajonc, Murphy, & Inglehart, 1989), makes one feel happier, either because the brain's electrical activity (Ekman & Davidson, 1993) or blood temperature (Zajonc, Murphy, & McIntosh, 1993) is affected by the action. These data suggest that putting on a happy face can actually improve one's mood.

   In a similar vein (so to speak), the changes in facial blood flow that cause blushing may increase embarrassment not just by complicating one's social predicament but by creating a real physiological feedback loop as well. In an automatic, unbidden process, the physical changes that accompany blushing may intensify one's emotional responses, regardless of the situation one faces. This view of blushing is held by Robert Edelmann (1987, 1994) of the University of Surrey, who believes that the mere act of blushing often makes embarrassment worse. Unfortunately, as Edelmann (1994) admits, there are not yet any data that conclusively support the feedback possibility, so it should merely be considered an interesting hypothesis for now. There is evidence that one's *beliefs* about one's physical reactions can influence the strength of one's embarrassment—using fake heart rate feedback, Shahidi and Baluch (1991) showed that young adults who believed their hearts were beating faster were more embarrassed after a conspicuousness manipulation than were those who believed their hearts had slowed—but we don't yet know whether blushing increases embarrassment in an automatic way that does not depend on the person's knowledge that he or she is blushing.

In any case, with its unusual vascular bed, the face does appear to be a site uniquely equipped to display a blush, and people are ordinarily born with a physiological capacity for blushing. Blushing appears to be a distinctive human capability. Still, not everyone blushes to the same extent.

## Who Is Prone to Blushing?

Blushing is often considered "the hallmark of embarrassment" (A. H. Buss, 1980, p. 129) but people do not always blush when they are embarrassed. Indeed, when they are later asked to recall their responses, people typically remember blushing in less than half of the embarrassments they encounter (Edelmann, 1990b). Many people probably blush more often than they think, but it does seem that embarrassment can occur without an accompanying blush, and there appear to be reliable differences among people in their susceptibility to blushing.

In fact, Mark Leary and Sarah Meadows (1991) of Wake Forest University have developed a Blushing Propensity Scale to assess such differences. The scale asks respondents to rate the frequency with which they blush in 14 different social situations. Some of these are clearly embarrassing circumstances, but, thinking that differences in blushing might be especially obvious in less threatening conditions, Leary and Meadows included several mundane situations as well. The entire inventory is reprinted in Table 8.1.

Average scores on the scale range from 30 to 45 for both men and women (Halberstadt & Green, 1993; Leary & Meadows, 1991). To the extent one's score on the Blushing Propensity Scale falls below or above that range, one tends to blush rather less or more often, respectively, than most people.

Interestingly, despite our stereotypes of "blushing brides"—and despite the fact that women are more embarrassable than men—women do not appear to blush more often than men do. There's no difference in their reports on the Blushing Propensity Scale, and there is no important difference between men and women when they are simply asked how often they blush (Shields, Mallory, & Simon, 1990). For instance, using a sample of 302 California college students, Angela

Simon and Stephanie Shields (1996) found that 52% of the women and a similar 44% of the men reported blushing at least once per week.

On the other hand, some individuals are clearly more prone to blushing than others. Embarrassability is closely related to blushing propensity, and highly embarrassable people do blush more often than other people (Halberstadt & Green, 1993; Leary & Meadows, 1991). There are other influential personality characteristics as well, including fear of negative evaluation and interaction anxiety, that is, the tendency to experience anxiety in social encounters even before anything goes wrong (Leary & Meadows, 1991). People who are chronically nervous

### TABLE 8.1. The Blushing Propensity Scale

How often do you feel yourself blushing in this situation? Please rate the frequency with which you blush in each of these situations, using the following scale:

    1 = I never feel myself blush in this situation.
    2 = I rarely feel myself blush in this situation.
    3 = I occasionally feel myself blush in this situation.
    4 = I often feel myself blush in this situation.
    5 = I always feel myself blush in this situation.

1. When a teacher calls on me in class.
2. When talking to someone about a personal topic.
3. When I'm embarrassed.
4. When I'm introduced to someone I don't know.
5. When I've been caught doing something improper or shameful.
6. When I'm the center of attention.
7. When a group of people sings "Happy Birthday" to me.
8. When I'm around someone I want to impress.
9. When talking to a teacher or boss.
10. When speaking in front of a group of people.
11. When someone looks me right in the eye.
12. When someone pays me a compliment.
13. When I've looked stupid or incompetent in front of others.
14. When I'm talking to a member of the other sex.

*Note.* From "Predictors, Elicitors, and Concomitants of Social Blushing," by M. R. Leary and S. Meadows, 1991, *Journal of Personality and Social Psychology, 60,* p. 256. Copyright 1991 by the American Psychological Association. Reprinted by permission.

in their interactions with others blush more readily than do those who are relaxed and comfortable when they socialize. Low self-esteem is also involved, so that those who tend to hold themselves in low regard blush more often than those with better opinions of themselves (Leary & Meadows, 1991).

Altogether, blushing propensity seems to resemble embarrassability in being based in an exaggerated concern with what others may be thinking that is blended with the fear that those judgments are negative. It seems to differ from embarrassability, however, in being a little more broadly based. Whereas embarrassable people dread the violation of social norms and react more strongly to them when they occur, people who are especially prone to blushing worry and fret about their interactions even when nothing untoward has occurred. The single best predictor of blush proneness *is* embarrassability, so that people who blush frequently do tend to react strongly to embarrassing circumstances. Another factor that augments their propensity for blushing and differentiates it from simple embarrassability, however, is chronic unease and nervousness in social situations.

This pattern is particularly evident among people for whom blushing is a dreaded component of ordinary interactions. *Chronic blushers* are plagued by unwanted blushing that occurs not because of some embarrassing incident, but simply because others are present. Any situation in which another person is a potential judge of their behavior may cause a blush in such people, making blushing a commonplace event that may occur several times a day. Two large groups of chronic blushers have been studied by Robert Edelmann (1990a, 1990b, 1991), who recruited his respondents when they wrote to request advice on coping with blushing that was advertised in a popular British magazine. On the whole these people were troubled by very frequent episodes of blushing; a male accountant (quoted in Edelmann, 1990a, p.12) wrote that he was likely to blush in

> "any situation which involves being with people. I hate going to places where there are a lot of people because I know I will blush. I even dread going to the doctor, dentist or seeing my children's teacher at school or even meeting old friends or relations who I have not seen for a while because I know I will blush."

Similarly, a young woman noted that she blushes "if I'm introduced to any new person or even buying something in a shop. Really any occasion where it is likely that people will notice/look at me" (Edelmann, 1990b, p. 218). Such people would no doubt report very high scores on the Blushing Propensity Scale!

Edelmann (1991) found that such chronic blushers were typically made so anxious by the prospect of interaction with others that they fit the psychiatric criteria for a diagnosis of *social phobia,* a powerful, persistent fear of situations in which one is exposed to scrutiny by others (American Psychiatric Association, 1994). In these extreme cases, a tendency to blush obviously transcends mere embarrassability, and is characterized by a global dread of social evaluation that pervades the person's social encounters. As a result, these chronic blushers often try to arrange their lives so that they can avoid contact with strangers. Whereas embarrassable people merely try to avoid embarrassing circumstances, people who are very prone to blushing often try to avoid other people altogether.

Happily, few of us are so afflicted. Such problems are not rare—perhaps 2% of American citizens, roughly 5,000,000 people, are burdened with social phobia (Marshall, 1994), for instance—but most of us are only moderately embarrassable and prone to blushing. Moreover, within that average range, blushing is ordinarily associated with events that are obviously embarrassing (Crozier & Russell, 1992). It appears that blushing may occasionally be a signal of broader concerns, but for most of us, most of the time, a blush is a sign that we're embarrassed.

A final point that may be reassuring is that, if you're not a chronic blusher, your tendency to blush may decline with age. In a study with a diverse group of teens and adults, Shields and her colleagues (1990) found that two-thirds of their younger respondents reported blushing frequently, at least once a week, but only 28% of those age 25 or older blushed that often. One reason for the decline may be a change in the blood vessels that allow blushing to occur; the neurochemical receptors that control the dilation of the facial veins become less numerous with time (Mellander et al., 1982). In addition, as people grow older and wiser, they may become less concerned with what others are thinking of them, causing both embarrassability and blushing propensity to drop with age. You may not be blushing as often 10 years from now as you do today.

## Are There Cultural Differences in Blushing?

In a series of studies, Robert Edelmann and his collaborators have asked 900 people across Western Europe (Edelmann et al., 1989; Edelmann & Neto, 1989) and Japan (Edelmann & Iwawaki, 1987) to think of a recent embarrassment and to recall whether or not they blushed. The remembered prevalence of blushing during these episodes was very similar from country to country—with 21% of the Spaniards, 25% of the Greeks, 29% of the Italians, 30% of the Japanese, and 34% of the West Germans reporting blushing—except in the United Kingdom, where 55% of the respondents recalled a blush. It's hard to know what to make of this. On the one hand, with the exception of the United Kingdom, there was an impressive similarity in the remembered frequency of blushing across different cultures. On the other hand, blushing may actually be much more common in some cultures, such as the United Kingdom, than others. The problem is that retrospective self-reports like these can be influenced by a variety of memory biases and normative expectations. It's possible, for instance, that blushing is simply a more salient component of an embarrassment prototype to people in the United Kingdom, leading them to notice or recall it more often even though it actually occurs at about the same rate.

The best conclusion at this point may be that there is some variation in the prevalence of blushing across cultures but that, on the whole, such differences do not appear to be too dramatic. (Obviously, that conclusion assumes that people in London really aren't blushing two-and-a-half times more often than people in Madrid.) Further support for this point of view comes from a comparison of the self-identified Asians, blacks, Hispanics, and whites in Simon and Shield's (1996) sample of California college students. There were no differences across ethnic groups in their reported frequency or duration of blushing, but blushes were much more visible on people with lighter skins than on those with darker complexions. Some of the differences in reported blushing across cultures may depend on the readiness with which blushes are noticed and remarked upon by others, and that probably occurs somewhat less often in more southern regions such as Spain, Italy, and Greece where people often have more swarthy skin.

In any case, people clearly blush all over the world, regardless of their skin color or culture (Leary et al., 1992). A change in skin color as a result of facial vasodilation may be harder to detect in dark-skinned peoples, but the capacity for blushing seems to be a human universal nonetheless. Moreover, as far as we know, Mark Twain was right: Humans *are* the only animals that blush. These facts point to the most interesting question about blushing of them all.

## Why Does Blushing Occur?

Our species seems to be equipped with a specialized physiology in one delimited region of the skin that allows involuntary, often visible vasodilation that does not occur elsewhere in the body. Why did Mother Nature go to the trouble to create such a response? As a starting point, it's usually safe to assume that nature is parsimonious and that such mechanisms are not frivolous extravagances; complex natural processes almost inevitably exist only because they are, or were once, useful in some way. This reasoning dates back to Charles Darwin and pertains to human emotions and emotional expressions, just as it does to other behavioral systems: "The reason the primary, prototypic emotions developed in the first place, were shaped and reshaped over the millenia, and continued to survive, was because they were adaptive" (Hatfield & Rapson, 1990, p. 129; also see Fridlund, 1994; Plutchik, 1980, in this regard).

As used here, "adaptive" means that an emotion was advantageous, improving a person's chances of surviving long enough to reproduce; it does not mean that the emotion was pleasant or desirable. Furthermore, emotions that were ordinarily adaptive may not have been valuable on all occasions; evolutionary theorists routinely acknowledge that a mechanism that is advantageous in one environment may not necessarily be beneficial in different circumstances (e.g., D. M. Buss, 1990). Indeed, to the extent that human culture has changed, mechanisms that were adaptive in our prehistory may not be advantageous at all today.

Thus in pondering the origins of an unusual but innate facial expression such as blushing, we need to recognize that times change more quickly than our species does. As Leary and Kowalski (1995) noted, "one must remember that our evolutionary ancestors spent most of the last several million years as foragers or hunter–gatherers, and that whatever psychological mechanisms evolved did so because of the evolutionary pressures under which these prehistoric beings lived" (p. 28). As a result, "all people are living fossils with complex design features that are records of prior selection pressures" (D. M. Buss, 1990, p. 282). It is possible, then, that blushing is merely an archaic response, an outmoded remnant of the past that has no useful function for anyone reading this book.

On the other hand, like other evolved emotional expressions, blushing may convey meaningful information about a person's mood and intentions that continues to be of use today. One recipient of such information is the person who is blushing, who, as we've seen, may gain some rough feedback about the extent of his or her own embarrassment. More importantly, emotional expressions can also be significant *interpersonal* signals that inform others of one's state (Oatley & Jenkins, 1992). According to emotion theorist Robert Plutchik (1980, p. 5), visible indications of a person's emotional state often "act as signals and preparations for action. They communicate information from one animal to another about what is likely to happen and thereby affect the chances of survival." Moreover, certain emotional responses fit Nico Frijda's (1986) definition of *interactive expressions*, which seem to exist primarily to influence the behavior of other people; these are expressions that are "shown for the sake of influencing others, appear to have developed for, or because of, such effect, and occur under eliciting conditions in which influencing others in that particular way appears to be of distinct instrumental value" (p. 25). Blushing is an imperfect gauge of the intensity of embarrassment (Leary et al., 1992), and it doesn't appear to serve any other valuable biological function, so it may well be an interactive expression that evolved because of its interpersonal effects.

Well, what effects are those? People are typically cowed by unwanted evaluative attention from others when they are blushing. They are usually conciliatory, often submissive, and rarely belligerent. A blush is also a guarantee that its owner cares about what others are thinking of him or her. Furthermore, blushes are involuntary responses that people cannot consciously control, so they cannot be faked or feigned; as a result, a blush is a trustworthy marker of a person's sensitivity to others' judgments. In short, blushing may be a reliable indication of a person's concern for social acceptance, and when it follows a clear social transgression, it may communicate a person's chagrin and regret about the event as well.

This point of view was eloquently expressed by Italian researchers Cristiano Castelfranchi and Isabella Poggi (1990), who suggested that

> those who are blushing are somehow saying that they know, care about, and fear others' evaluations and that they share those values deeply; they also communicate their sorrow over any possible faults or inadequacies on their part, thus performing an acknowledgment, a confession, and an apology aimed at inhibiting others' aggression or avoiding social ostracism. (p. 240)

A blush may thus be a sincere *nonverbal apology* for past or possible misbehavior that informs others of one's genuine contrition and desire to avoid rejection (Semin & Manstead, 1982). By blushing, people may plainly signal their pain at a violation of shared norms and may communicate their distress over making an unwanted impression; the blush may also convey their eagerness to make amends.

In fact, some observers have always considered blushing to be a measure of a person's social and moral conscience. For Darwin and his contemporaries, "blushing showed the spiritual and moral side of human nature more clearly than any other facial display. Only blushing, it was thought, could prove that men and women had a conscience, that they could tell right from wrong and feel guilty when they overstepped the boundaries of convention" (Browne, 1985, p. 317). Similarly, in 1910, Havelock Ellis asserted that a capacity for blushing could distinguish civilized people from lesser types: "Inability to blush has always been considered the accompaniment of crime and shamelessness. Blushing is also very rare among idiots and savages" (p. 138).

The obvious consensus is that blushing communicates bona fide sensitivity, gentility, and apologetic chagrin to observers, which allows the provocative possibility that blushing evolved in the first place because of its adaptive interpersonal effects. Strategies for making amends and seeking atonement for misdeeds are needed by all human cultures (Eibl-Eibesfeldt, 1989), and blushing may be an interactive expression that became common among our ancestors just because it helped fulfill those ends. By reassuring others who may have been doubtful of one's moral or social competency, blushing may have decreased the chances of the abandonment or rejection that would have been catastrophic to our forebears. If so, blushing would have had real survival value, and people who blushed would have had an evolutionary advantage over those who did not blush. Over time, blushing would have become ingrained in our species, even if it gradually became less useful as an interpersonal signal among equatorial peoples whose skin grew darker as an adaptation to the sun (cf. Leary et al., 1992; Simon & Shields, 1996).

One answer to the question of why people blush, then, is that blushing is an evolutionary adaptation that serves the need to belong. As a universal, involuntary signal of chagrin and concern over social evaluation, blushing helps placate potential critics of one's behavior and forestalls social rejection; people who blush are presumably less likely to be snubbed and shunned following some public predicament than are people who do not blush.

This is a fascinating idea, but, as an alert reader, you may have noticed that I have yet to mention a shred of actual research evidence that supports it. Indeed, let's be cautious here; it would be remarkable if a physiological reaction that (1) is often aversive, and (2) makes people even more conspicuous when they're already fretful about undesired social evaluations, actually had desirable interpersonal effects. Let's also remember that blushing is just one of several nonverbal reactions that may demonstrate that someone is embarrassed, and observers' judgments may be influenced by these behaviors as well. So, we still need to determine definitively whether blushing helps to mollify and appease others when we transgress. However, the answer may involve other signs of embarrassment as well.

## GAZE AVERSION, SMILE CONTROLS, SHEEPISH GRINS, AND OTHER SURE SIGNS OF EMBARRASSMENT

Even if people don't blush, they can certainly look embarrassed. Whether or not a blush is present, embarrassment is ordinarily accompanied by specific nonverbal behavior that appears to reliably indicate that a person is, in fact, embarrassed. However, unlike other emotional expressions that can be captured in a single static "snapshot" (such as happiness, which is denoted by a smile and crinkling of the skin at the side of the eyes), embarrassment is communicated by a particular *pattern* of body and facial movements that make it distinct.

One exacting analysis of the sequence of facial actions that accompanies embarrassment was conducted by Dacher Keltner (1995) of the University of Wisconsin. Keltner scrutinized videotapes of young adults who were performing a variety of awkward tasks in a psychology lab; when they said they were embarrassed, Keltner examined the individual action of specific muscle groups in their faces using a research tool known as the Facial Action Coding System (Ekman & Friesen, 1978). Embarrassed people did several things differently than those who were, for instance, merely amused by their unusual tasks.

First, embarrassment was characterized by *gaze aversion*. When abashment struck, people looked away from others, typically shifting their gaze to the left and then looking down more quickly and for a longer period than they did when they were pleasantly amused. (Curiously, when amused people did look elsewhere, it was more often to the right than to the left.) Embarrassed people also had restless eyes; while they continued to avoid eye contact with others, they shifted their gaze from place to place more frequently than did those who were not embarrassed.

Then, literally a split second later, embarrassed people typically began trying to control emerging smiles with cheek and lip movements called *smile controls*. These were epitomized by attempts to pull down the corners of one's mouth, and biting or pressing one's lips together in order to minimize or obscure an imminent smile. Embarrassment was accompanied by quicker smile controls, and a greater number of smile controls, than amusement was.

Ordinarily, these efforts were only partially successful because most, though not all, people then exhibited a *smile* shortly thereafter. On the whole, these were not smiles of genuine amusement; they were noticeably less intense than the smiles displayed by happy people, and seemed to be nervous, silly, self-conscious grins rather than indications of honest delight (see Leary et al., 1992). In fact, in his own investigations, Jens Asendorpf (1990) has demonstrated that embarrassed smiles can be reliably distinguished from smiles of real mirth by the timing of the gaze aversion that accompanies the smile. When people are embarrassed, they look away from others 1½ seconds before their smiles reach their broadest, fullest points. (Keltner [1995] observed this, too.) In contrast, when people are genuinely amused, they usually look away ½ second *after* the broadest expanse of their smiles. The two patterns are clearly different, and a mixed message is evident in the embarrassed pattern; as Asendorpf noted, "embarrassed smiles carry the flavor of ambivalence: approach (smiling) and avoidance (gaze aversion) at the same time" (1990, p. 102).

Indeed, once they had smiled, most embarrassed people lowered their heads and turned them away, more often to the left than to the right (Keltner, 1995). These *head movements* were also avoidant gestures, and they were often followed with the last facial sign of embarrassment, a *face touch* by a hand that further obscured a smile or hid the eyes. A lowered head was about three times more likely during embarrassment than amusement, and a face touch was more than twice as likely to accompany embarrassment as mirth.

Altogether, this sequence of embarrassed responses usually occurred in the order described above, over a period of just a few seconds. On average, gaze aversion began $7/10$ of a second after embarrassment struck, and ended, along with some final gaze shifts and head movements, 5 seconds later. Naturally, individuals' responses could be idiosyncratic, and not everyone exhibited all of these behaviors. Still, there was impressive uniformity in individuals' displays of embarrassment; almost half of Keltner's embarrassed participants displayed a prototypical pattern consisting of—in order—gaze aversion, smile controls, and head movements, and almost none of those who were simply amused behaved this way.

With all of these cues available, audiences could reliably distinguish embarrassment from amusement just by watching people's faces (Keltner, 1995). However, Robert Edelmann and Sarah Hampson (1981b) have found that embarrassment is even easier to detect if observers can see people's bodies, too. Edelmann and Hampson prepared videotapes of embarrassed or amused people from the neck up, from the neck down, or from the neck up *and* down (this last version being an unedited tape of each person's entire face and body). People engage in more nervous *body motion* when they become embarrassed, shifting their posture, moving their legs and feet, and gesturing with their hands (Edelmann & Hampson, 1979, 1981a), and when these data were combined with facial information in Edelmann and Hampson's study, a person's embarrassment was especially plain to anyone who happened to be watching.

A soundtrack can be helpful, too. When they induced embarrassment in young adults through staged awkward interactions, Edelmann and Hampson (1979, 1981a) found that people made more *speech errors* when they were embarrassed than they did when all was well. They hesitated clumsily, stuttered, stammered, mispronounced words, and generally misspoke more often after they became embarrassed than they had before. All of these are indications of a nervous lack of poise, and people's embarrassment was evidently apparent in their voices as well as on their faces.

Finally, there is one last sign of embarrassment that is not perceptible to others but that may be influential, nonetheless. When embarrassment strikes, people may feel *physical symptoms* of their emotional arousal that affect their experiences. When Denny Fahey and I asked college students who had performed some embarrassing tasks to rate some specific sensations, they told us that they experienced more muscle tension, more "butterflies" in their stomachs, higher heart rates, and, of course, warmer cheeks than did other students who had not been embarrassed (Miller & Fahey, 1991). They were absolutely right on at least one count; we actually measured their cheek temperatures and found them to be significantly warmer than those of their nonembarrassed counterparts. Thus embarrassment can be accompanied by a variety of internal sensations in addition to blushing that may provide meaningful signals to the embarrassed person (cf. Edelmann, 1990a; Pennebaker & Roberts, 1992). Only one of these symptoms, increasing cheek temperature, may be unique to embarrassment but several systemic changes can occur (Leary, Rejeski, et al., 1994), and they may be dramatic enough on occasion to affect the person's judgments of the intensity of his or her embarrassment.

Increased heart rate and muscle tension were also deemed to be signs of embarrassment by Edelmann's (1990b) international respondents, and did not differ substantially across cultures. Indeed, the various nonverbal behaviors described above tended to characterize embarrassment around the world.

## USING THE SIGNS

If you knit all of these nonverbal behaviors together into one 5-second sequence, you get a fairly dramatic tableau. What's more, the pattern formed by these responses conclusively indicates that a person is embarrassed. Keltner (1995) found that embarrassment could be accurately distinguished from amusement, enjoyment, anger, disgust, and shame using these cues, and he concluded that embarrassment was typified by a recognizably distinct facial display all its own. Other displays may be similar, but no other set of interpersonal signals is quite the same. Gaze aversion and head movements downward are also common when people experience shame, for instance, but smile controls and face touches are conspicuously lacking. In fact, Keltner found that when the prototypical elements of gaze aversion, smile controls, head movement, and face touches were all present, embarrassment was correctly identified by observers an impressive 92% of the time.

Furthermore, keep in mind that none of this depends on the presence of a blush. Even if blushing isn't visible, embarrassment may be obvious; add a noticeable blush and it may be positively unmistakable. Our measurements of the cheek temperatures of students who were performing embarrassing tasks indicated that the stronger their blushing, the more embarrassed they said they were and the more embarrassed they appeared to others (Miller & Fahey, 1991). As you'd expect, blushing is yet another useful guide to the apparent severity of someone else's embarrassment.

Altogether, the coherent timing of this nonverbal sequence (Asendorpf, 1990; Keltner, 1995) also suggests that the signals of embarrassment are far from being chaotic or disorganized. We may certainly *feel* flustered and bewildered when embarrassment strikes, but our actions may be much less erratic than our thoughts. Viewed from start to finish, a nonverbal display of embarrassment may be complex and animated, but orderly, nevertheless (Heath, 1988). As unplanned and reflexive as it may be, embarrassed behavior fits a recognizable pattern that can make it a clear, consistent signal of its owner's embarrassed state.

Importantly, this all means that when we are embarrassed, others are likely to know it. These various signals can combine to provide a *reliable interpersonal communication* that embarrassment has occurred, regardless of who's embarrassed or who's watching. We're all unique people and our embarrassments may be weak or strong, but some embarrassments can be glaringly obvious to everyone present.

My colleagues David Marcus, Jeff Wilson, and I explored this issue in a study that examined the interpersonal perception of embarrassment in groups of young adults (Marcus, Wilson, & Miller, in press). We invited female students at Sam Houston State University to attend lab sessions in groups of five, and then had each, in turn, perform a series of either embarrassing or innocuous tasks as the other women watched through a one-way window in an adjacent room. This procedure meant that each participant watched all of the others perform the tasks and was watched by them as well; then, each woman described how embarrassed she believed each of the others had been. This elaborate method allowed us to determine the parts played in the communication of embarrassment by each woman (each "actor") and her audience. If the recognition of embarrassment depended on the idiosyncratic decoding skills of the members of the audience, a particular woman's embarrassment would be perceived differently by the various people watching; an actor's apparent embarrassment would be in the "eye of the beholder" because different beholders would differ in their judgments of the same event. On the other hand, if the diverse audience members *agreed* in their judgments of how embarrassed someone was, embarrassment would apparently be obvious on the face of the beheld, being so plain as to leave little room for disagreement among different observers.

We found that strong embarrassment was, in fact, obvious. When the women performed the embarrassing tasks, there was little variability in the judgments of those who were watching. Strong embarrassment was plainly evident in the face and actions of the embarrassed person, no matter who she was, allowing anyone watching to realize the extent of her chagrin.

In contrast, there was much more idiosyncrasy in the communication of weak embarrassment; there, both the actor's and audience's personalities were influential. The women who performed the more innocuous tasks did nothing very daunting but they did know that others were watching, and some (but not all) became mildly embarrassed. In such cases, there was significant disagreement among the watchers in the next room about how embarrassed each actor was, and in both instances—both looking mildly embarrassed and recognizing mild embarrassment in others—an individual's embarrassability was key. Highly embarrassable actors looked more embarrassed and their embarrassment was easier to detect. In the audience, more embarrassable watchers recognized embarrassment in others that cooler observers did not notice. Thus, people seemed to differ in their display and recognition of mild embarrassment, whereas strong embarrassment was more universally understood. Whether *your* audiences notice your mild embarrassments may depend on your susceptibility to embarrassment and on just who's watching; on the other hand, if you become quite embarrassed, your chagrin and abashment will probably be obvious to everyone present.

These data allow the possibility that displays of embarrassment really are interactive expressions that are meaningful communications that can have substantial influence on others. Embarrassment is certainly recognizable, which must be true in order for blushing and the other signs of embarrassment to be useful nonverbal apologies for public transgressions. *Are* they unspoken apologies? If we can judge by how others respond when they detect embarrassment in others, the answer, remarkably, is "Yes."

## HOW OTHERS REACT

We have arrived at one of the more amazing, really intriguing truths about embarrassment. As goofy, awkward, and uncomfortable as it feels, it can have desirable interpersonal effects. If we have made an unwanted impression, if we have violated others' reasonable expectations and embarrassment is a normal response to the situation, *others will like us and treat us better if we do become embarrassed* than they will if we remain unruffled, cool, and calm.

This assertion may be surprising because we dislike embarrassment and avoid it whenever we can. Indeed, embarrassment only becomes appropriate when we have failed to conduct ourselves or our interactions properly, and are already facing an unwanted predicament. However, *given that a predicament has occurred,* embarrassment ordinarily appears to be an adaptive, useful response to adverse social situations that helps to minimize the interpersonal damage that results.

Several studies support this point. They show that embarrassment is more likely to elicit acceptance and approval from others than it is to rouse rejection and disapproval. Audiences really do respond to embarrassed actors as if they (the actors) had already apologized for their misdeeds. British researchers Gün Semin and Tony Manstead (1982) demonstrated this when they showed undergraduates at the University of Sussex videotapes of a male shopper accidentally knocking over a big display of toilet paper rolls in a grocery store. Four different tapes were prepared. In one version, the fellow became obviously embarrassed but walked away from the spill and simply continued shopping. In a second tape, he left the scene without appearing embarrassed at all. In the other two versions, however, the shopper patiently rebuilt the display and repaired his accidental damage, appearing embarrassed in one tape and cool and calm in the other. The observers' evaluations of the shopper revealed that someone who made restitution without obvious chagrin seemed especially mature. In contrast, someone who remained unruffled but who did not make amends was judged to be particularly unreliable and unlikable. Across the board, however, the fellow was liked better when he was embarrassed by his mishap than when he was not. Someone who became embarrassed and repaired the damage was very well liked, of course, but even the fellow who just walked away in evident mortification received somewhat kinder judgments than someone who made restitution with unflustered aplomb.

The student observers in Semin and Manstead's (1982) study simply watched another person's predicament, but the adults participating in an investigation by Edelmann (1982) were actually involved in someone else's plight. Edelmann's procedure induced participants to give another person very negative feedback about his performance on a task. They had to tell the fellow face to face that he had done very poorly, and they did this not knowing that he was an accomplice of the experimenter who was carefully trained to react in one of three ways. In one condition, the accomplice reacted to the distressing news with an implacable, defiant stare. In another, he acted rather embarrassed by averting his gaze, fidgeting, and making speech errors, and in a third condition, he acted even more embarrassed by adding smiling and laughter to the gaze, body, and speech cues. The participants' liking for the accomplice and their own comfort with the interaction were then assessed, and once again, obvious embarrassment engendered positive responses. The accomplice was liked more when he was obviously embarrassed than when he was not, and the participants were more at ease during the difficult interaction, too. As in Semin and Manstead's study, apparent embarrassment elicited kindly, approving reactions from others instead of disapproval and rejection.

Parents may even punish their children less severely when they misbehave if the children appear embarrassed, rather than unperturbed, by their actions. Semin and Papadopoulou (1990) presented mothers with a vignette of a child dropping and breaking a bottle of juice at a grocery store, and then asked them how they would respond and how embarrassed their own children would be in such a situation. The more embarrassment the mothers expected from their children, the less punitive their own reactions were expected to be. Just as Castelfranchi and Poggi (1990) proposed, embarrassment seemed to deflect and defuse criticism and correction that the parents would otherwise provide.

These investigations all suggest that signs of embarrassment really do help mollify observers who might otherwise form less desirable impressions of the embarrassed person, and they support the possibility that embarrassment serves as a nonverbal apology for untoward events. Embarrassment is not a panacea, however. Exaggerated embarrassment that completely incapacitates a person and disrupts a situation further may make a relatively poor impression on others. Levin and Arluke (1982) had a young woman ask for help with a research project in several college classes, and had her make the request in one of three ways. In one case, she performed smoothly, describing her project and distributing sign-up sheets without incident. In contrast, in a second case, she dropped her pile of sheets on the floor and picked them up in a nervous, flustered manner before proceeding with her appeal. In a final condition, she dropped the sheets and became so upset that she blurted, "Oh, my god! I can't continue," and scurried out of the room. (The classes' instructors then passed out the sheets for her.) Interestingly, the students volunteered considerably more help to the woman when she flubbed and then recovered than they did when she did not become embarrassed at all. Mild embarrassment that briefly interrupted, but did not destroy, the interaction elicited kindly support from the audience. On the other hand, the observers provided almost no help whatsoever to the woman when she became so flustered that she had to flee.

Apparently, embarrassment that supports the possibility that a person's predicament is a temporary, distressing aberration makes a better impression than does embarrassment that reinforces the presumption that one is unduly inept. Embarrassment seems to elicit favorable reactions from others when it *improves* an unwanted image, presumably by communicating that the embarrassed person finds his or her misdeeds to be surprising, uncustomary, and disquieting. Erving Goffman (1956) asserted this very point when he argued that embarrassment serves the desirable function of demonstrating that, while the embarrassed person "cannot present a sustainable and coherent self on this occasion, he is at least disturbed by the fact and may prove worthy at another time" (pp. 270–271). On the other hand, embarrassment that seems overblown may make matters worse by portraying the embarrassed person as oversensitive, clumsy, and timid. In order to make the best possible impression on others, given that an unwanted predicament has occurred, the best advice may be: all things in moderation. Remaining too cool in the face of untoward events may portray one as crass and unfeeling, but becoming too flustered may portray one as inept. Remarkably, however, appropriate, moderate embarrassment elicits approving reactions from others, making a person seem more likable than he or she seems when such embarrassment is not present.

## Pratfall Effects

This potential benefit of embarrassment may be surprising, but other similar effects exist. If one is well respected, simply getting into an embarrassing predicament in the first place can improve one's overall image. Desirable people who accidentally commit physical pratfalls are sometimes liked better after such incidents than they were before. In one study of this effect, Aronson, Willerman, and Floyd (1966) asked college students to listen to a tape of a fellow student auditioning for a quiz show. In one version of the tape, the contestant did very well, correctly answering nearly all of his difficult questions. In a second version, the contestant did similarly well but then noisily spilled coffee over his new clothes. Listeners were asked for their evaluations, and they actually liked the successful contestant better when he committed the blunder than when he didn't.

I think that I've encountered examples of this myself. As a college professor, I occasionally do or say things in front of large classes that are so embarrassing that my audiences laugh at me. My missteps *are* embarrassing, but afterwards I'm often secretly glad that they occurred. They provide information about me that is inconsistent with my desired identity of a sage, mature authority, but as long as I respond with moderate, appropriate embarrassment, they also demonstrate that I'm a normal guy with a good sense of humor. Usually (because of my hard-won experience with such events), audiences get to see me handle the event with humility and self-deprecating humor but then quickly recover my poise and get on with the class. In such cases, I fail to manage the usual professor role appropriately but otherwise do pretty well, and I think most of those embarrassments are endearing, not demeaning; they improve our rapport.

On the other hand, this may all depend on whether my classes think well of me in the first place. Pratfalls only have desirable effects when one is already liked and respected by one's audience. If a person already seems unskilled or incompetent, a pratfall is not endearing at all. Aronson et al.'s (1966) study also had some listeners hear tapes in which the contestant did poorly; he got only 30% of the questions right, and spilled the coffee in one version but committed no such blunder in another. The mediocre contestants were liked less than the superior contestants were, and they were liked least of all when they spilled the coffee. A predicament that humanized and improved the identity of a superior candidate harmed the identity of a mediocre person, who may have seemed simply inept.

Thus, I caution you against actually creating your own intentional embarrassments to improve your public image. First, the generality of the pratfall effect is a bit uncertain. Studies of the effect have only examined physical pratfalls and inept performances, so we can't be sure that other types of embarrassing predicaments have the same effects. In addition, most of us tend to overestimate how likable and competent we are (S. E. Taylor & Brown, 1988), so it might be dangerous to assume that we're so well respected that pratfalls would help! Finally, the effect may hold for only some observers or only in some cases. Helmreich, Aronson, and LeFan (1970) demonstrated that people of average self-esteem found the blunders of superior people to be endearing, but audiences who had high self-esteem did not. The effect may depend on whether the pratfall makes one seem more similar or more dissimilar to one's audience.

Nevertheless, the possibility that embarrassing events can ever endear us to others is potentially important. Embarrassment can be a dreadful experience, but the research evidence argues that it often really is less awful than it may seem. Not only do signals of embarrassment often elicit favorable responses from others, but our predicaments themselves may seem more humorous and endearing to others than we think. The pratfall studies again suggest, as Levin and Arluke's (1982) study did, that embarrassing events can be either demeaning or charming depending on how we respond to our predicaments. If we get moderately embarrassed but then laugh at ourselves, or apologize, thereafter smoothly regaining our poise, we may seem reasonably competent and more likable *because* a predicament occurred. However, if we get so flustered that we cannot regain our poise and the interaction is ruined, our exaggerated embarrassment may make us appear inept and leave an audience with a negative impression despite our evident chagrin. We'll return to this idea in Chapter 9; for now, let's again note that embarrassing events may often be less fearsome and humiliating than they sometimes seem. In addition, our responses to a given predicament may play a key role in determining whether an episode of embarrassment is ultimately awful or endearing.

## Appeasement in Primates

Several signs of embarrassment bear an interesting resemblance to the stereotypic behaviors with which nonhuman primates, such as chimpanzees and baboons, deflect social threats from other members of their groups (Leary & Kowalski, 1995). A steady look from another animal is a sure sign of assertion or aggression in these species (Bolwig, 1978), and when confronted in this way, a lower-status animal typically lowers its gaze and bares its teeth in a mirthless, sheepish grin (Van Hooff, 1972). These are apparently gestures of appeasement because the dominant animal ordinarily looks away, mollified, when they are displayed (Goodall, 1988).

Similar steady staring from others often causes embarrassment in humans, and Mark Leary (1995; Leary & Kowalski, 1995) speculated that it is no accident that gaze aversion and silly smiling are also signs of embarrassment. Just as in nonhuman primates, the function of these signals may be to appease other people; indeed, they may have become reliable signs of embarrassment because they successfully do so. Leary noted that the appeasement grins of chimpanzees are remarkably like the sheepish human smiles that accompany embarrassment, and as we have seen, such signals typically do engender favorable responses from observers. Thus it may be that a baboon's appeasement displays and our embarrassed behavior share similar origins; both may have evolved to protect social inclusion (and physical well-being) during episodes of social threat.

Admittedly, this is a very speculative notion. Nevertheless, the similarity of the behaviors lends some credence to the idea that embarrassment serves functions such as those that motivate appeasement displays in other animals (Castelfranchi & Poggi, 1990), and I think it's fascinating that nonhuman primates behave much as we do in these situations when it is advantageous for them to do so.

## Wanting Others to Know We're Embarrassed

Embarrassment is uncomfortable, and we avoid it when we can. However, if obvious embarrassment really does reassure observers of our good nature after some minor transgression, we probably should not try to hide our embarrassment from others. To the contrary, we should probably be glad that our audiences *do* know of our embarrassment, and should express it to them if it is not already evident. Mark Leary, Julie Landel, and Katharine Patton (in press) examined this daring notion in two studies at Wake Forest University. In a first investigation, Leary et al. asked students either to listen carefully to or to sing along with a taped version of the song "Feelings" with an experimenter in the room. (Devilishly, the researchers admitted that they picked that tune because it makes even good singers sound silly.) Singing the song was pretty embarrassing, and, afterwards, the students were allowed to express how embarrassed they had been in one of three ways. Some participants handed explicit ratings of their embarrassment to the experimenter, who inspected them closely. Other participants completed similar reports but then stuffed them in a sealed box out of the experimenter's view. Finally, a third group made no reports at all and were given no opportunity to describe, even to themselves, how embarrassed they had been.

At this point, then, some participants had been embarrassed by a foolish task and knew that the experimenter was aware of their chagrin, while others were just as embarrassed but had not explicitly expressed it to anybody. The students were then asked to complete another questionnaire that, they were assured, would be carefully examined by the experimenter. Those who had not yet communicated their chagrin to the experimenter now reported considerably more embarrassment than those who had already expressed their chagrin. Moreover, those who had previously informed the experimenter of their embarrassment were now no more embarrassed than those who had never been very embarrassed at all (having merely listened to "Feelings" without singing it). Knowing that their audience was aware of their embarrassment seemed to reduce the severity of their predicament, diminishing the embarrassment they felt. Meanwhile, those who had never made their embarrassment plain seemed to remain motivated to express it.

In a second study (Leary et al., in press), the experimenter asked participants to sing "Feelings" into a tape recorder privately, but then embarrassed some of them by playing the tape. During the excruciating playback, the experimenter casually told some students that they seemed to be blushing, but did not mention a blush to others. Afterwards, the students were asked for various self-ratings, and, in an apparent attempt to repair their damaged social identities, those who believed that they had not been seen blushing conveyed more positive impressions of themselves to the experimenter than did those whose blushes had been noticed. Having no blushes to help remediate their predicaments, the nonblushers seemed to turn to other means to avoid rejection by the experimenter. In contrast, those whose blushing was acknowledged described themselves in ways that were no different from participants who had never been embarrassed in the first place; with a blush in place, no other response seemed to be needed to overcome their predicaments.

Remarkably, these results suggest that recognition of one's embarrassment by one's audience can actually reduce one's distress. The data don't necessarily demonstrate that those whose embarrassment is unacknowledged are actually more eager to make their embarrassment known to others, but, given the apparent ameliorative effects of obvious embarrassment, perhaps they should be. In Leary et al.'s studies, those whose embarrassment was recognized by others acted as if their predicaments were past, or had never happened at all. Here, as in other studies of the signals of embarrassment, obvious embarrassment seemed to serve a remedial function of helping to repair, rather than exacerbate, awkward situations and unwanted evaluations.

## CONCLUSIONS

Embarrassment is ordinarily accompanied by a distinctive pattern of nonverbal behavior that makes it a readily recognizable emotion. Furthermore, as long as one's embarrassment is not exaggerated or unduly disruptive, observers typically respond to a display of embarrassment with more, not less, liking for the embarrassed person. No study has yet examined how observers judge someone who becomes embarrassed in the *absence* of any predicament, so we should not assume that embarrassed behavior is inherently likable. Instead, it is probably helpful because it communicates a person's real distress, abashment, and chagrin to others and, by so doing, reassures those others that an *undesired* impression has been conveyed by the person's prior actions.

What makes this possibility especially intriguing is how unexpected it is. Most people seem to be unaware of embarrassment's potential benefits as a healing response to unwanted events; when they are embarrassed, people typically expect the worst, and sometimes react in ways that ensures they get it. Motivated by embarrassment, people often behave in conciliatory, desirable ways, but they occasionally make their problems much worse, as we'll see in the next chapter.

# CHAPTER 9

# *Responses to Embarrassment*

If we misunderstand embarrassment, it's not from lack of experience. College students are embarrassed more than once a week, on average (Stonehouse & Miller, 1994), and embarrassment is one of the emotions that is mentioned most frequently in routine conversation (Shimanoff, 1984). With all this attention and practice, you might think that most people would be seasoned pros at deftly handling embarrassing predicaments, but of course that's not true. Collectively, we're clueless about what to do when embarrassment strikes, a failing that may be rooted in several important misperceptions.

First, people usually consider embarrassing circumstances to be worse than they really are. Embarrassed people commonly fear that they have done more damage to their social identities and made poorer impressions on others than they really have. A series of studies by Gün Semin (1982) and Tony Manstead (Manstead & Semin, 1981; Semin & Manstead, 1981) demonstrated this point nicely. They asked German or British college students to consider various predicaments either from the perspective of an observer watching someone else do something embarrassing, or from the position of the actor who was actually doing it. Among other examples, "observers" were asked to consider someone who is seen picking her nose, or spilling a pint of beer on a stranger in a crowded pub, or ripping his pants during intermission at a play, while "actors" imagined being caught picking their noses, ripping their pants, and so forth. Across the diverse misdeeds, actors consistently believed they had conveyed a more negative image of themselves to others than the observers said they did. The observers were routinely more forgiving than the actors thought they would be.

One reason why people overestimate the harm done by social predicaments is that they don't appreciate the value of appropriate displays of embarrassment. Most people haven't read Chapter 8, and don't know that obvious embarrassment routinely elicits liking instead of disapproval from others. I observed this misunderstanding myself when I asked students at Sam Houston State University to forecast what would happen when they became embarrassed. In that procedure (Miller, 1988), participants learned that they would soon perform Apsler's (1975; see Chapter 3) embarrassing or innocuous tasks while another student watched from an adjacent room. Before the tasks, however, I asked them to predict what the observers would think of them after their performances. Those facing the daunting, embarrassing activities feared the worst; they thought they would look foolish to the observers and they expected to be disliked. They were quite wrong. Those who performed the embarrassing tasks did become embarrassed, but they were liked *better* by their audiences than were those who performed the more mundane, innocuous tasks and who were never embarrassed at all. Once again, appropriate embarrassment engendered liking, and as in Semin and Manstead's (1981; Manstead & Semin, 1981) studies, people miscalculated the interpersonal harm done by an embarrassing predicament.

A final important misunderstanding is that many people probably believe that they dread embarrassment and go out of their way to avoid it more than other people do. There's a good reason for this: When we feel cowed by the threat of embarrassment and quietly change our behavior to avoid potential conspicuousness or chagrin, our personal fear of embarrassment is often very salient. However, when other people do comparable things, we typically fail to recognize that a similar fear of embarrassment is at work. We are familiar with our own efforts to avoid embarrassment but rarely detect them in others. As a result, we may come to feel that we are more uneasy about embarrassment than others are. Dale Miller[1] and Deborah Prentice (1994) suggested that this sort of thing often occurs in college classrooms (and other group meetings). After an especially obtuse lecture, a professor will ask if there are any questions. The students in the audience will have dozens of questions but may be reluctant to ask the first question because of a nervous wish to avoid becoming conspicuous. In such a case, when no one asks any questions, each individual is likely to be painfully aware of the dread of embarrassment inhibiting his or her own behavior, but is likely to assume—wrongly—that the classmates just didn't have any questions. The result is that embarrassment feels more fearsome to us than it appears to be to most others.

Feeling unduly cowed by embarrassment and overestimating its harm (as well as underestimating its value) can make embarrassment seem less manageable and more intimidating than it rightfully is. As a consequence, people may inconvenience themselves or even risk real harm in order to avoid trivial embarrassments, and they may react to unavoidable predicaments in maladaptive, unhelpful ways. This is often needless. In this chapter, I describe how people react to embarrassment, both as embarrassed actors and as witnesses of others' embarrassments. I think you'll find that, as in the preceding chapter, an important conclusion emerges from several studies: Embarrassment's not as bad as most people think it is.

## AVOIDING EMBARRASSMENT

People dislike embarrassment and avoid it when they can, doing so in at least two different ways. One means is to avoid others' scrutiny when a predicament is anticipated or has already occurred. For instance, when college students know that they will soon be embarrassed, they avoid contact with others. Given a choice, they prefer to be alone (Fish, Karabenick, & Heath, 1978; Friedman, 1981) or they favor others who ignore them (Ellsworth, Friedman, Perlick, & Hoyt, 1978). This is interesting because some negative emotions actually promote affiliation with others; when people are fearful, for example, they eagerly seek others' company (Fish et al., 1978). This tendency is the basis for the cliché, "misery loves company," but as Fish et al. noted, "some types of misery (embarrassment) do not prefer *any* type of company" (p. 264). Because embarrassment is necessarily a public event, people seek solitude when it is imminent.

If a predicament has already occurred, people will conceal it if possible, even when it is costly to do so. As we discussed in Chapter 1, Brown (1970) demonstrated that college students will forego tangible profits in order to keep others from learning of their embarrassing behavior. In Brown's study, keeping an embarrassment quiet was more important to the students than were the cash payments they could have received by describing it to others. Furthermore, the more intense the embarrassment (Brown & Garland, 1971) and the more judgmental the audience (Garland & Brown, 1972), the greater the sacrifices people made to avert disclosure. Obviously, the more severe their predicaments, the more motivated people are to evade unwanted attention.

A second, more provocative means of avoiding embarrassment is to change one's behavior to prevent a predicament from happening at all. People often make small alterations in their actions to avoid failures of privacy regulation, abashed harmdoing, conspicuousness, and various other types of embarrassing circumstances. When these are trivial adjustments involving little cost or effort, they are often amusing or simply polite. For instance, Lewittes and Simmons (1975) planted unobtrusive observers in a college bookstore and found that men were likely to purchase a few additional items, such as another magazine or candy, when they were buying a *Playboy* or *Penthouse* magazine, but they tended to get just the magazine if they were buying *Time* or *Newsweek*. Of course, by buying several items the men were able to avoid the mildly embarrassing perception that they had come into the store just to get the Pet of the Month. What they didn't know was that the cashiers were cooperating with the study, and had been told not to bag a fellow's purchase unless he specifically requested it. As you'd expect, the men rarely asked for a bag for *Newsweek*, but they usually asked for a bag for *Playboy*. Overall, the study demonstrated the subtlety with which people sometimes fine-tune, and occasionally conceal, their behavior to forestall embarrassment.

Unfortunately, our modest efforts to avoid embarrassment are not always innocuous. People often fail to perform small kindnesses for others that they would readily render in situations that did not create some threat of embarrassment. In one example, researchers arranged for a young woman to drop, apparently by accident, either a box of envelopes or a box of tampons directly in the path of a man or woman walking behind her (Foss & Crenshaw, 1978); she then continued walking, ostensibly unaware of her loss. Three-fourths of the men retrieved the envelopes for her, but they picked up the tampons only a third of the time. Obviously, many men decided not to help the woman—and just to leave the tampons lying on the ground—when they saw what the box contained. In contrast, women were as likely to retrieve the tampons as the envelopes, presumably because the tampons were less embarrassing to them. However, when McDonald and McKelvie (1992) staged a similar event with a mitten or a box of condoms, neither men nor women were as likely to pick up the condoms as they were the mitten.

In these studies, people were clearly willing to be deliberately unhelpful in order to avoid a potentially awkward interaction. Of course, it's one thing to fail to help others and quite another to punish *oneself*, but people will also inconvenience themselves to avoid embarrassment. Druian and DePaulo (1977) told Vassar College students they were doing poorly on a difficult test, and then gave them the opportunity to ask for aid from a competent helper who was said to be either a child or a fellow adult. Although it meant they would continue to struggle, the students asked for less help when it would come from the child than they did when help would come from a peer. In this case, maintaining the right public image was evidently more important than doing well on the test.

The examples cited thus far are trivial, but they allow the more important possibilities that people may occasionally (1) fail to help others who desperately need it, or (2) do themselves meaningful harm, in order to avoid unwanted evaluations from mere strangers or acquaintances (Leary, Tchividjian, & Kraxberger, 1994). In emergencies, people who would have acted had they been alone may stand by and do nothing when other witnesses are present because of their fear of becoming embarrassed (Latané & Darley, 1970). In too many other instances, people sacrifice their own long-term well-being in order to evade temporary, short-term embarrassment (Leary, 1995; Leary & Kowalski, 1995). It's regrettable, but "the emotional desire to avoid embarrassment . . . [can] motivate irrational and even self-harmful choices" (Baumeister & Scher, 1988, p. 11). For instance, sexually active teenagers may fail to use any contraception during intercourse, even though they know it's risky, because they think it will be embarrassing to obtain contraception from a physician or pharmacy (Herold, 1981; Leary & Dobbins, 1983). People who desire safe sex and who even have a condom in a purse or pocket will fail to use it because they think it will be embarrassing to negotiate its use with their partners (Helwig-Larsen & Collins, 1994; Hobfoll, Jackson, Lavin, Britton, & Sheperd, 1994). In medical situations, women will avoid needed mammography (Lerman, Rimer, Trock, Balshem, & Engstrom, 1990) and pelvic exams (Kowalski & Brown, 1994), men will avoid prostate exams (Leary & Kowalski, 1995), and everybody will be reluctant to mention the alcohol and drug use, cholesterol intake, smoking, emotional problems, and lack of exercise their physicians need to hear (Leary & Kowalski, 1995). Those who need psychotherapy may be too embarrassed to get it (M. Weiner, 1992), and people may even quietly choke to death in a crowded restaurant rather than make an embarrassing scene (Heimlich & Uhley, 1979). Obviously, "the yoke of embarrassment is so strong that people sometimes do things contrary to their own or others' best interests to avoid being embarrassed" (Leary & Kowalski, 1995, p. 99).

This is truly the dark side of embarrassment. Perhaps, as Arnold Buss (1980) proposed, some of our cultures rely too much on embarrassment as a tool of socialization, so that, after years of teasing and ridicule from parents, teachers, and peers, many of us fret overmuch about the possibility that total strangers will get an unwanted impression of us. On the other hand, we need to note that while a collective desire to avoid embarrassment can have individual costs, it also has societal benefits. On the whole, people seeking to avoid embarrassment are likely to attend and adhere to desirable social norms, being less nosy and more considerate, polite, respectful of others, charitable, honest, lawful, and careful than they otherwise would be (e.g., Fiske, 1993; Grasmick,

Bursik, & Kinsey, 1991). In this fashion, a drive to avoid embarrassment can be a desirable agent of social control throughout our lives, encouraging each of us to be steadfastly moral and respectable (Kemper, 1993).

The key may be to allow embarrassment to have the useful effect of steering us toward desirable behavior without letting it push us into maladaptive, unhelpful, injurious conduct. We'll consider how this may be done in Chapter 10. For now, however, we can draw an important conclusion about social life: For many of us, a quiet but compelling drive to avoid embarrassment pervades our daily activity. As Mark Leary and I noted elsewhere, "the possibility of being embarrassed seems to dictate and constrain a great deal of social behavior; much of what we do and, perhaps more important, what we don't do is based on our desire to avoid embarrassment" (Miller & Leary, 1992, p. 210).

## RESPONDING TO EMBARRASSMENT

Nevertheless, despite our efforts, none of us is a stranger to embarrassing predicaments.[2] Sooner or later, we normal folk find ourselves mortified and chagrined by unwanted events that threaten to portray us to others in undesired ways. Once we find ourselves in a predicament, there are several different things we can do, ranging from the planful to the panicky and from the conciliatory to the antagonistic (Cody & McLaughlin, 1985). Our possible responses also differ in the likelihood that they will help restore a desired public image; although a response to embarrassment has to fit the situation in order to be successful (M. B. Scott & Lyman, 1968), some responses are generally more helpful in regaining an audience's trust and respect than others.[3] Unfortunately, one of the simplest responses is also one of the least helpful: taking flight.

### Flight

People sometimes become so thoroughly mortified by an embarrassing event that they simply flee the scene with no explanation (Cupach & Metts, 1990; Froming et al., 1990). When such a physical retreat occurs, people end an encounter abruptly and leave in haste and obvious disarray. This rarely seems to be a thoughtful, considered response to a predicament, and instead suggests that the person is overwhelmed. Barry Schlenker (1980) presumed that flight was most likely when one's embarrassment was intense, one's expectations of successfully coping with the circumstances in some other manner were low, and the possibility of escaping others' surveillance was high. The problem, of course, is that flight often just delays one's troubles and can be counterproductive later on. "In fact," noted Schlenker, "it can turn the predicament from bad to worse" (p. 135). It leaves audiences with a poor impression (Levin & Arluke, 1982), portraying the fleeing actor as inept and flighty (if you'll pardon the pun), and that can exacerbate one's difficulties if one ever encounters that audience again. It is certainly a simple reaction—just run!—but is quite panicky, is mildly antagonistic (harming rather than improving one's relation to the audience), and usually hurts, rather than helps, one's image. We can usually do better.

## Evasion

Another straightforward response is to ignore the embarrassing event. With evasion, an embarrassed person simply does not acknowledge his or her predicament and tries to act as if nothing has happened (Cupach & Metts 1990; Metts & Cupach, 1989).[4] This can be done deftly or awkwardly. A clumsy variant of evasion is to allow the predicament to interrupt one's activity while nonetheless remaining silent and offering no explanation or apology. This form of evasion is ungainly because the interaction grinds to a halt and one simply does nothing about it; one's embarrassment gets the upper hand. In one example of this (see Miller, Bowersox, Cook, & Kahikina, 1996), a young woman was enjoying a pleasant conversation with a classmate when she committed a cognitive error, addressing the classmate by the wrong name; flustered, she stopped talking, but offered no other response. She did not explain her brief lapse and tried to let the matter drop, but did so awkwardly and at the cost of the ongoing interaction.

Used more skillfully, evasion allows someone to gloss over an embarrassing event as if it had never happened; the embarrassed person quickly regains his or her poise and the interaction continues largely unabated, with no mention of the untoward event. Indeed, evasion can be a very graceful response to minor embarrassments. When a predicament is ignored, the embarrassed actor implies that the undesired event is of little note and can be swiftly forgotten; better simply to overlook it than sidetrack the proceedings with an elaborate apology or befuddled chagrin. As Bill Cupach and Sandra Metts (1994) note, belaboring a minor infraction often creates more inconvenience for all concerned than it resolves. Thus, when someone shrugs off embarrassment quickly and chooses not to acknowledge the event, evasion is moderately planful and makes a somewhat positive impression, but is neither particularly conciliatory nor especially antagonistic (lying near the midpoint between the two); in being evasive, the person neither seeks forgiveness from the audience nor heeds the possibility of its rebuke. This sort of indifference is a handy way to get past small mishaps. However, it is clearly inappropriate after more major transgressions; a person who seems fairly nonchalant about his or her glaring deficiencies does not make a good impression at all.

## Humor

A response that acknowledges one's predicament but treats it lightly is humor (Edelmann, 1982; Fink & Walker, 1977). Unlike evasion, humor admits that unwanted events have occurred. However, like evasion, making a joke or laughing at oneself implies that one's transgression is relatively trivial, needs no explanation, and can be readily overcome. It informs the audience that the embarrassed actor considers his or her predicament to be manageable and that he or she is capable of continuing the interaction, but it also communicates the actor's specific wish to regard the situation as comedic rather than grave.

For that reason, like evasion, it is undoubtedly better fitted to some circumstances than to others. Some social situations in which norms are broken are inherently comical, whereas others are irritating and aggravating (Argyle, Furnham, & Graham, 1981). Robert Edelmann (1982, p. 366) suggested that when the audience is not harmed and no serious rule is broken, humor can "alleviate discomfort in two main ways: first, it may act as a tension reducer" for everyone present, and second, "laughter by the embarrassed person allows the other interactant[s] to laugh back." Indeed, audiences may often be uncertain whether an event is silly or serious until it is defined for them by the actor's response to the event. Consider a woman falling off some stairs into a cluster of people at a relatively formal party: If she says, " 'Hi, I just thought I'd drop in' " (Metts & Cupach, 1989, p. 156), the situation is obviously less serious and probably less awkward for the audience than if she makes a flustered apology or says nothing at all. (On the other hand, a wry quip is completely out of place if she injures someone else in her fall.) Humor is usually more planful than evasion because one must think of something to say, and it is probably perceived to be more conciliatory, but it resembles evasion in making an impression that is only somewhat positive.

## Accounting

On other occasions, people not only acknowledge their predicaments, they try to explain them to others, providing *accounts* that are designed to reduce the apparent severity of their transgressions (Schlenker, 1980; Schönbach, 1990; M. B. Scott & Lyman, 1968). There are two different types of accounts; both are very planful, but they differ in how conciliatory they are (Cody & McLaughlin, 1985) and in the global impressions they make on others (Riordan, Marlin, & Kellogg, 1983).

## Excuses

When people offer excuses, they try to shift some of the blame for an unwanted predicament someplace else, reducing their apparent responsibility for the embarrassing events. There are two general ways to do this. People can claim that the events were unintended and/or uncontrollable ("I didn't mean it"; "I didn't want this to happen") or that extenuating circumstances were at fault (" 'I couldn't help it, I was drunk . . . coerced . . . under strain . . . too turned on to stop . . . tired . . . a victim of an impoverished environment,' and so on" [Schlenker, 1980, p. 142]). In either case, people seek to deflect some of the social disapproval that might accompany their predicaments, and, as long as their excuses are reasonable, they are usually successful (Gonzales, 1992; Riordan et al., 1983; B. Weiner, 1993). Ducking some of the blame with a good excuse typically makes a better impression on an audience than taking the blame and trying to justify one's actions to others.

## Justifications

With a different kind of account, people accept the responsibility for a predicament but assert that it's not so bad, downplaying the negative ramifications of the event. There are various ways to justify embarrassing behavior (Schlenker, 1980), but none of them are particularly conciliatory. People can claim that their predicaments are not as severe as they first appeared ("It's only a small stain") nor as severe as others in the past ("At least it wasn't the guacamole again"). Alternatively, they can suggest that a predicament actually has hidden benefits that make it worthwhile ("I bet she'll buy stronger picnic plates next time"). Such justifications often succeed in reducing observers' appraisals of the severity of a predicament (Riordan et al., 1983), but they're not very effective at eliciting forgiveness from others (Cupach, Metts, & Hazleton, 1986). People who justify their transgressions are judged to be guilty of lesser crimes, but they're seen as guilty nonetheless. There's a better way to take the blame.

## Apologies

When people offer apologies, they accept responsibility for their predicaments, sometimes specifically citing their culpability, but they also seek atonement. A minimal apology may be a perfunctory request for forbearance ("Excuse me"),[5] but full-blown apologies can include expressions of remorse and regret ("I'm so sorry"), fervent pleas for forgiveness ("Please forgive me"), self-castigation ("I'm so clumsy sometimes"), offers of restitution ("Let me make it up to you"), and promises of better behavior in the future ("I'll never do it again") (Schlenker & Darby, 1981). Nevertheless, whatever their form, good apologies fulfill two valuable functions in addition to admitting blame: They *"redress the past* and they extend a *promise of more desirable conduct in the future"* (Schlenker, 1980, p. 155). When they follow embarrassing predicaments, good apologies communicate an actor's desire to distance him- or herself from the untoward events, and they ask the audience's absolution. Apologies are very conciliatory, and they make a favorable impression on others (Cupach et al., 1986). There are times, however, when they're all talk and no action.

## Remediation

Because apologies only *offer* restitution, Metts and Cupach (1989; Cupach et al., 1986) found it useful to distinguish verbal apologies from actors' actual attempts to repair or redress any damage or disturbance stemming from their predicaments. People often try to clean up their spills, zip up their zippers, and compensate others for their inconvenience, and while verbal apologies often accompany such actions, behavioral remediation can occur without explanation or apology. Such efforts can be either frantic or deliberate, but they are implicitly conciliatory, and they make much better impressions on others than do responses that leave one's damage for others to repair (Semin & Manstead, 1982). Remediation is akin to a nonverbal apology, conceding one's responsibility and repairing the problem, and is almost diametrically opposed to responses to embarrassment that aggress against others.

## Aggression

Physical or verbal attacks against others only rarely follow embarrassing predicaments, but they are possible (Cupach & Metts, 1992). Aggressive responses almost never occur unless one's predicament is the result of audience provocation, with embarrassment resulting from someone else's meddling, teasing, or practical joke. However, when they do occur, aggressive responses are antagonistic, further disrupting the situation, and they make a poor impression (although the aggressive actor is unlikely to care very much). Anger and hostility are less likely when one's embarrassment appears to have been accidentally provoked by others, but more likely when one's embarrassment seems to have been

intended by others (Martin, 1987; Sharkey, 1992), unless the provocation was expected as part of an accepted ritual.

## Compliance

A last response to embarrassment is also infrequent, but is worthy of
mention as a counterpoint to aggression. On occasion, people are
intentionally embarrassed by others, and they merely comply with the
others' behavior, passively allowing themselves to be a conspicuous
and/or laughable target. Such responses tend to occur as part of various
rituals that follow a predictable pattern, such as wedding or baby showers
in which an engaged couple or expectant parents are feted with gifts and
celebration; the participants often *expect* there to be some mischievous
teasing of the honored guests. Dawn Braithwaite (1995) observed several such events and found that their games and activities were often
intended to be playfully embarrassing. For example, in one case a
blindfolded groom was asked to feel the hands of several women to find
the hands of his fiancée, and in another a 40-year-old father-to-be was
asked to diaper a baby doll in front of his enthusiastic colleagues with a
timer running and an audiotape of a crying baby playing loudly. The
most common response to such situations was cheerful, if reluctant,
compliance, even though the events were often quite embarrassing. Of
course, in these cases, compliance is conciliatory and makes a good
impression, and Braithwaite noted that "embarrassing acts may not be
perceived as negative by a recipient when the *context* dictates the
appropriateness of embarrassment" (p. 155). Her point is an apt re-
minder that selection of a response to embarrassment should be guided
by the nature of one's predicament.

## SELECTING A RESPONSE

Back in 1955, when he was formulating his theory of impression management, Erving Goffman used the term "face" to describe a person's
desired social identity, or the image that a person seeks to establish in
the eyes of others. The term caught on, and in one way or another, all
of the responses to embarrassment described above can be said to be
examples of *facework*, verbal and nonverbal coping actions meant "to
overcome feelings of embarrassment in an attempt to regain social
composure and the smooth flow of interaction" (Edelmann, 1994, p.
232). Good facework repairs and restores the desired public images of
both the embarrassed actor and anyone else who may have been affected
by the predicament, but that definition makes it clear that not all efforts

to "save face" after an embarrassing event are equally efficacious. For instance, Marvin Scott and Stanford Lyman (1968) suggested that successful facework must be both reasonable and adequate, fitted to the gravity of one's offense. "Reasonable" responses to embarrassing predicaments fit the facts as they are known to the audience; claiming "I was pushed!" as an excuse for a pratfall when there was no else nearby would obviously be absurd (and, being incredible, would create a even bigger threat to face). "Adequate" responses fit the severity of a predicament; as noted earlier, a pratfall that only wounds one's dignity can be laughed off, but humor would not be appropriate if anyone is really injured. Thus, the suitability of the various responses to embarrassment can depend on the exact nature of one's predicament, as can one's *desire* to engage in facework in the first place.

## The Facework Motive

People are not equally motivated to redress all of the predicaments they encounter. First, we care more about some audiences than others (Leary, 1995), and our motive to save face after some adverse event will ordinarily depend on our current desire to make a certain impression. As I suggested in Chapter 7, embarrassment hinges on our concerns about what others are thinking of us; as a result, if a person really doesn't care how a particular audience judges him or her, even an astonishing transgression would not be very embarrassing, and little facework would result. Of course, most of us care (perhaps too much) what total strangers think of us, so we usually try to save face no matter who's watching. Nevertheless, we're likely to try harder in front of important audiences whose evaluations really count.

Our facework motives are affected by the severity of our predicaments as well. Events that do greater damage to our desired identities or that have more adverse impact on other people offer more formidable self-presentational dilemmas (Cupach, 1994; Schlenker, 1980). In particular, as our behavior becomes increasingly offensive or does more actual harm to others, more elaborate and conciliatory responses are required if face is to be restored (Schlenker & Darby, 1981). Marti Hope Gonzales and her colleagues at the University of Minnesota demonstrated this with an ingenious laboratory procedure that induced students to ostensibly do either minor or grievous harm to a fellow student (Gonzales et al., 1990). Participants in the study appeared to knock a cup of cola—which was actually controlled with an invisible wire—off a table into the other student's tote bag, which turned out to contain either a damp computer printout or an expensive, ruined camera and flash. As you'd expect, the hapless participants were more apologetic when they had done more harm. In general, severe predicaments seem to engender more fervent facework (Modigliani, 1971; Schlenker, 1980).

Once it is aroused, the desire to save face can be powerful and enduring. It can be worth more than money. Bert Brown (1968) placed college students in a bargaining simulation in which they could either act cooperatively and maximize their profits or dominate the other player at the expense of their own earnings. The simulation was supposedly conducted with an audience watching, and in its first phase, the participants were always exploited by the other player (who was part of the research team). Thereafter, the participants received word from the audience that they had either "looked good" for playing fair or "foolish and weak" for being exploited, and the simulation resumed. Those who believed they had not lost face chose to maximize their earnings, having no reason to do otherwise. In contrast, those who had been embarrassed by the other player retaliated against him in a show of strength, even though they lost money by doing so. Reestablishing a desired image for the audience appeared to be valuable to these people, who sought to save face even when it was costly to do so.

The motive to regain lost face can even outlast the situations that create it. Robert Apsler (1975) embarrassed students at Boston University by having them perform several foolish tasks (e.g., dancing to recorded music; imitating a 5-year-old throwing a temper tantrum) in front of a fellow student. Then, either the observer or a third person (both of them part of the research team) who did not know about the embarrassing performance asked the participants for help with a class project. The embarrassed participants generously offered more help than did other, unembarrassed students who had performed some innocuous tasks, and they did so regardless of who asked. Once embarrassed, they seemed to have a general motive to seek social approval, pursuing it even from another person who was completely unaware of their recent predicament. Thus, people were not completely free of the effects of a prior embarrassment when they entered a subsequent interaction with a brand new audience, and embarrassment did not affect only the situation in which it occurred. Instead, until lost face was restored, facework continued even when the predicament was past. Facework often ends quickly once it seems to succeed, but if people remain uncertain about their acceptance by others, it may persist for some time (Leary et al., in press).

## The Choices People Make

When the facework motive is aroused, what responses do people select? This is no simple question; the choice of a response to embarrassment may be quite idiosyncratic. Not only may it depend on the severity of the predicament, it may change with the importance of the interaction, the relative status of those involved, and the intimacy the actor shares with his or her audience (among other factors; see Cody & McLaughlin, 1985). As one example, humor may be more common among equals than among those who differ in status, where it can be misconstrued as laughing *at* rather than *with* someone (Fink & Walker, 1977). Furthermore, high-status people are less likely to apologize for small transgressions than are those of lesser prestige (Gonzales et al., 1990).

Moreover, when they are flustered and emotional, people may not always make the most sensible choice. Karen Leith and Roy Baumeister (in press) threatened college men with embarrassment by asking them to sing the audacious song "My Way" into a tape recorder held for them by a female experimenter. As they considered this daunting request, they were also asked to make a choice between two lotteries, one of which offered a very good chance of winning a small ($2.00) award, and another that offered an almost nonexistent chance of winning a much larger ($25.00) award. Importantly, the men also learned that if they didn't win the money they'd have to listen to a loud 3-minute tape of fingernails screeching across a blackboard. This made the $25 lottery a risky, irrational choice, but almost all (87%) of the men facing embarrassment selected that option, whereas fewer than half (40%) of the men in a neutral control group made that choice. Leith and Baumeister argued that, in the throes of a negative emotion such as embarrassment, people become more impulsive; they seem "to seek out the best possible outcome and grab for it, without being deterred by rational cost–benefit calculations or even by the prospect of possible unpleasant consequences" (p. 34).

Thus, people may not always be coolly logical when embarrassment strikes. On the other hand, many of the responses people make to their actual predicaments seem fairly reasonable. Several studies have examined responses to embarrassment either by asking people to evaluate various possible reactions to a particular predicament (Cupach et al., 1986; Petronio, 1984) or by asking them to describe what they actually did during a recent embarrassment (Cupach & Metts, 1992; Metts & Cupach, 1989; Sharkey & Stafford, 1990). In one instance, using the latter procedure, Kathy Bowersox, Richard Cook, Christine Kahikina, and I analyzed 257 accounts of embarrassment from students at Sam Houston State University and found obvious differences in the frequency with which the assorted responses were used (Miller et al., 1996). Our results are listed in Table 9.1. Across diverse predicaments, the most common response was evasion; more than a fourth of the time, people tried to go on as if nothing had

**TABLE 9.1. Actors' Responses to Their Embarrassment**

| Response | Frequency of use |
|---|---|
| Evasion | 28% |
| Remediation | 17% |
| Humor | 17% |
| Apology | 14% |
| Flight | 9% |
| Excuses | 8% |
| Aggression | 5% |
| Justification | 2% |
| | 100% |

happened, ignoring the predicament or quickly changing topics of conversation. Quite a few embarrassments were never explicitly acknowledged by the actor involved.

On most occasions, however, embarrassment clearly altered the trajectory of an interaction, either being specifically addressed or ending the interaction altogether. Out of every 11 embarrassments, 1 resulted in the actor taking flight and running away, but remediation was more common, occurring in nearly a fifth of all predicaments. People were more likely to try to correct the cause of their problems than simply to flee them. Indeed, if verbal apologies and remediation are considered together, close to a third of the embarrassments were answered with some sort of effort to atone for one's actions.

In contrast, people seldom tried to justify embarrassing actions. Justifications were used rarely. Excuses were employed more often but still infrequently, so that one or the other form of accounting occurred only 10% of the time. On the whole, remediation and apologies that redressed undesired conduct were much more frequent than accounts that merely excused or justified such actions.

Humor (in a tie with remediation) was actually the second most common individual response, occurring in one of every six embarrassments. People were much more likely to wryly acknowledge their difficulties than to try to excuse them. Moreover, humor was far more prevalent than aggression.

Importantly, various studies also show that certain responses are more likely to follow some incidents than others. Apologies and remediation are particularly likely after any event that inconveniences other people, such as abashed harmdoing or failures of privacy regulation (Cupach & Metts, 1992; Sharkey & Stafford, 1990). Justifications almost never occur after such events (Cupach et al., 1986), but are more typical in episodes of conspicuousness (in which people really are not guilty of any obvious rule violation and evidently wish to announce their innocence). Excuses often follow cognitive errors, but humor is rare in such situations; instead, humor is especially common after physical pratfalls and various losses of control (Cupach & Metts, 1992; Metts & Cupach, 1989). Finally, aggression occurs only in cases of audience provocation (Metts & Cupach, 1989; Sharkey & Stafford, 1990). Even though embarrassment is an uncomfortable emotion, it almost never fosters hostility toward others unless those others are the cause of one's embarrassment. As we suggested in Chapter 2, this is one of the telling differences between embarrassment and shame; shameful people tend to be surly and antagonistic toward others (Tangney, 1995). Embarrassed people may often evade mention of their plights or flee them altogether, but embarrassment also routinely motivates conciliatory behavior de-signed to win renewed approval from others (Apsler, 1975; Metts & Cupach, 1989).

I should also note that people may respond to a given predicament in more than one way. Cupach et al. (1986) found that people used more than one response after a third of their embarrassments, stringing together two or more discrete tactics in an elaborate sequence of facework. Most of these sequences combined apologies with remedia-tion—so that people both asked forgiveness and cleaned up their messes—but various other combinations were possible. Other popular combinations paired apologies with humor or flight.

Overall, these patterns that link certain responses to particular predicaments seem sensible; for instance, it is more reasonable for humor to be employed when one is laughable, after a public pratfall, than it is when others are annoyed and an apology is called for, and that's just how people react. Nevertheless, it is interesting that such prudent patterns exist; they support a point offered by Heath (1988), who argued that, despite the flustered awkwardness of embarrassment, our responses to social predicaments are usually more organized and coherent than they sometimes seem to be. We certainly feel at a loss when embarrassment strikes, and our responses to embarrassing circumstances may not be calculated and contemplative, but they are often perfectly reasonable and adequate. Despite our possible impulsiveness (Leith & Baumeister, in press), our choices of responses do seem to be guided by the situations we face in a practical, rational way.

In fact, those choices do not seem to be much affected either by the intensity of a person's embarrassment or by that person's individual embarrassability. People who are very embarrassed tend to respond to their chagrin in the same way as those who are less emotional (Sharkey & Stafford, 1990), and people who are quite susceptible to embarrassment behave much like those who are less prone (Cupach & Metts, 1992). (This latter finding is another intriguing point about embarrassability; highly embarrassable people don't encounter different types of predicaments as anybody else [Miller, 1992], and they don't seem to respond differently to them, they are just more intensely affected by them [Miller, 1995b].) Men and women do differ in their expressed preferences for some of the strategies, however. Women think apologies and excuses are more helpful in overcoming embarrassment than men do, whereas men find evasion and humor to be more beneficial than women say they are (Cupach et al., 1986; Petronio, 1984). Indeed, when they did someone else harm in Gonzales et al.'s (1990) study, women offered longer, more explicit apologies than men did. Nevertheless, both sexes consider apologies to be more effective responses to embarrassment than excuses, justifications, or evasion, and, overall, there are no substantial differences between men and women in the ways they actually respond to particular predicaments (Cupach et al., 1986).

On the whole, then, people typically seek to regain their poise and ensure their social inclusion when they respond to embarrassment. On some occasions, they are either so overwhelmed that they abandon the scene and flee, or so aggravated that they stay and retaliate against those who caused their predicament. More often, however, they try to minimize the impact of unwanted events by ignoring or glossing over them, or—even more likely—acknowledging and then explaining them, remediating them, or apologizing for them. Most of these are rather conciliatory, agreeable actions that appear to be motivated by a desire to mollify suspicious or critical observers.

In fact, embarrassment may motivate people to adopt congenial social identities before it even occurs. In one of my studies (Miller, 1988), I warned college students that they would soon be embarrassed and then gave them a chance to introduce themselves to the strangers who would be watching them. Those facing an upcoming embarrassment were more modest, humble, and self-effacing than were those who did not expect to be embarrassed, and they actually made better first impressions. Those who did not anticipate embarrassment were more vain, and did not come across as well. Thus, although embarrassment is uncomfortable and can be accompanied by obnoxious behavior, this does not occur often, and most of the time when we're embarrassed, we are contrite, humble, and eager to please. Embarrassment typically motivates good-natured behavior.

## THE REACTIONS OF OTHERS

Of course, other people often do something about our embarrassments, too. Sometimes, they don't have much choice. Embarrassing predicaments can be problematic for everyone in the vicinity for several different reasons. First, because the signals of embarrassment can be so plain, others are likely to know that we're embarrassed (see Chapter 8), and, even from a distance, they may experience some empathic embarrassment (Miller, 1987, 1992). It is often affecting to witness someone else's humiliation; as Goffman (1956, p. 265) noticed, "when an individual finds himself in a situation which ought to make him blush, others present usually will blush with and for him" even if he doesn't have enough sense to blush on his own account. In addition, even if others remain unembarrassed, they may have to deal with our flustered chagrin. As established above, embarrassment usually changes the situations in which it occurs. Ongoing interactions may be sidetracked or entirely derailed to deal with a predicament, and even innocent bystanders may feel obliged to acknowledge a stranger's embarrassment in some way. Both the mortified actor and his or her entire audience may find themselves involved in remediating and overcoming an embarrassing incident.

Because of this, people are often motivated to avoid *others'* embarrassments as well as their own. They avoid delicate topics of conversation, lower their blinds, soften their criticism, and refrain from mentioning others' transgressions to keep from embarrassing someone else. On occasion, others may even deftly save us from embarrassment without our knowledge. Rom Harré (1995) provided such an example: When a waiter at an exclusive restaurant was asked by an unsophisticated patron (who was hoping to impress his clients) to make sure their dry, red wine was cold, the waiter quietly replied, "I'm terribly sorry, sir, the refrigerator's full. We'll have to serve it at room temperature." Because no one else noticed the exchange, the waiter's clever response nicely averted a potential predicament, and the patron wasn't even aware of the help he had received.

On other occasions, actors may enter into explicit agreements with their audiences that specify how they will collaborate to save face and avoid embarrassment. A woman of my acquaintance grew up in a home that had only one bathroom. Because both she and her father liked to linger in the bathtub in the evening, one of them often needed to retrieve something from the bathroom while the other was soaking in the tub. They agreed that, in order to avoid embarrassing violations of privacy, the person in the tub would close his or her eyes before inviting the other person to come in. This meant that the person in the nude was the one with eyes closed, so it didn't really protect anybody's privacy at all, but the violation was less noticeable that way, and they were content.

In fact, once a predicament has already occurred, our audiences frequently respond with similar cooperation and grace. Metts and Cupach (1989) asked their respondents what other people said or did during a recent embarrassment, and found that observers responded with a variety of tactics much like those available to the embarrassed actors themselves. Audience members did not often take flight, but they did offer various accounts on behalf of the actor, react with humor, pretend not to notice the actor's predicament, help clean up the damage, and sometimes chide the actor for unbecoming conduct. Thus, nearly all of the responses to embarrassment described thus far were used by bystanders as well.

### Empathy and Support

Importantly, most of the things observers did *helped reduce* an actor's embarrassment. Indeed, in two of every three embarrassments, observers responded in a fashion that helped the embarrassed actor regain his or her composure and resume the interaction (Metts & Cupach, 1989). The most common of these reactions was *support*. Observers often explicitly reassured the mortified actor of their continued positive regard for him or her, communicating their acceptance of the person despite the predicament. Embarrassed actors would get a quick hug or a pat on the knee and be advised, "You're okay; don't fret over it."

The second most likely helpful response was *empathy*. Audiences often assured actors that their embarrassment was not unusual or uncommon, saying they were familiar with such predicaments (e.g., "I know how you feel; it happens to me all the time"). Altogether, as Table 9.2 shows, embarrassed people received either empathy or support quite often; on more than half of the occasions in which audiences were helpful, one of the two tactics was used. Moreover, when audiences opted for more than one response and combined two or more tactics in a remedial sequence—as happened about a third of the time (Cupach & Metts, 1990)—a combination of empathy and support was more likely than any other. Audiences almost never used a sequence of responses that did not include one or the other of these two.

### Humor

Humor was also a fairly frequent response. Audiences sometimes responded to a person's predicament with smiling or laughter that actually

TABLE 9.2. Observers' Responses to Others' Embarrassments

| When audiences were *helpful*, they used these responses: | this percent of the time: |
|---|---|
| Support | 32% |
| Empathy | 19% |
| Humor | 16% |
| Evasion | 12% |
| Justifications | 9% |
| Excuses | 7% |
| Remediation | 5% |
| | 100% |

| When audiences were *unhelpful*, they used these responses: | this percent of the time: |
|---|---|
| Humor | 38% |
| Attracting attention | 36% |
| Criticism | 21% |
| Doing nothing | 5% |
| | 100% |

*Note.* From "Situational Influence on the Use of Remedial Strategies in Embarrassing Predicaments," by S. Metts and W. R. Cupach, 1989, *Communication Monographs, 56,* p. 158. Copyright 1989 by the Speech Communication Association. Reprinted by permission.

made the person feel better. In such cases, the audience's good humor was not demeaning; instead, it probably demonstrated that they were taking the situation lightly instead of considering it to be a grave matter requiring serious attention. In this manner, humor can be a desirable response from an audience, minimizing rather than increasing the severity of one's predicament. Imagine inadvertently but loudly breaking wind in an elevator and having your fellow passengers either chuckle and smile at you or remain stonily silent, looking disgusted; which would you prefer?

Humor is a risky strategy, however; it "combines criticism with support, acceptance with rejection" (Coser, 1960, p. 91), and the recipient may not always be sure how to interpret it. Well-meant humor may not always be perceived to be supportive and sympathetic by the recipient. Indeed, when an audience's reaction does make someone's embarrassment worse instead of better, it is more often with humor than with any other response (Cupach & Metts, 1990). Thus, because of its potential ambiguity, the only safe laughter may be reciprocal laughter; Edelmann (1994) noted that laughter works best as a remedial strategy when both the actor and the audience respond with good humor. If only one or the other laughs, humor is less likely to help the actor overcome his or her embarrassment.

## Evasion and Other Responses

After support, empathy, and humor, evasion was the most frequent helpful response from observers. Audiences sometimes pretended not to notice someone's predicament and continued to behave as if no infraction had occurred. For instance, evasion was likely after an actor's cognitive error, with others failing to correct an obvious slip of the tongue, and it was especially common when an embarrassed actor used evasion, too (Sharkey & Stafford, 1990). If a person chose not to acknowledge his or her embarrassing miscue, the audience rarely brought it up.

Audiences occasionally offered justifications and excuses on behalf of an embarrassed actor, as well. They minimized the damage done, or explained why a predicament could have befallen anybody (e.g., "Those steps are slippery"). Such responses may have been particularly welcome because excuses work best when they are believed and accepted by one's audience (Doherty & Schlenker, 1995), and excuses suggested *by* the audience obviously fill the bill.

## Making Embarrassment Worse

Clearly, audiences often cooperated in helping embarrassed people reduce their chagrin. They were not always successful in doing so, however, and sometimes they didn't try. Cupach and Metts's (1990) respondents also recalled that other people did something that actually made an embarrassment *worse* about a third of the time. When audiences were unhelpful, their most frequent response was humor, as Table 9.2 shows. In some of these cases, the observers' good cheer was probably meant to be friendly and supportive, and was simply misconstrued; on other occasions, however, actors were jeered at and ridiculed by unsympathetic audiences.

The second most common unhelpful response called attention to the embarrassed actor's plight, potentially attracting a larger audience. Once again, some of these actions were not meant to add to the person's problems (look back at the example of "inadvertent disclosures" in Chapter 4), but others *were* intended to attract wider publicity. Douglas

Glick of Washington and Lee University once told me (personal communication, October 4, 1993) of his attempt to order a meal in Hebrew at a restaurant in Tel Aviv: Meaning to order a salad with "olives," he actually ordered a salad with "penises." Not only did his waiter laugh heartily, he yelled to all the kitchen staff, had them come out, and made Glick repeat his request! As Cupach and Metts (1990) noted, calling this sort of attention to an actor's behavior was often playful, but it was also one way audiences could implicitly chide the actor for misconduct.

Other efforts to reproach someone were more direct. Audiences sometimes scowled at an embarrassed actor, looking obviously displeased, or spoke up and criticized the person's inappropriate behavior. Of course, these actions confirmed an actor's fear that others were disapproving of him or her. However, it was also possible for actors to read disapproval into a total lack of response from an audience; on rare occasions, people became more embarrassed when observers failed to exhibit any reaction whatsoever. In such cases, audiences did not appear to be evasive, they seemed to be disinterested, and that lack of concern increased an actor's chagrin.

Thus, audiences weren't always helpful. Sometimes they bore no ill will toward an abashed actor but failed to communicate their support adequately. In other instances, they either made their disapproval clear or took obvious pleasure in the person's predicament. Even worse, as you may recall from Chapter 4, audiences sometimes intentionally acted to *create* a person's predicament in the first place.

### Intentional Embarrassment

Some of the embarrassments we encounter are caused by other people who *try* to embarrass us, usually with excessive teasing. Stonehouse and Miller (1994) found that 7% of our embarrassments are planned by others, and it's true that audiences often have selfish or spiteful intentions in mind when they produce them. William Sharkey (1992) asked more than a thousand people about occasions in which they had tried to embarrass someone else, and found that their intentions were unfriendly in such cases half the time. In close to 40% of intentional embarrassments, people meant to punish others by embarrassing them, either to get them to follow the rules or to retaliate against them for some past sin. This kind of intent was more common in schools (Martin, 1987) and in the workplace (Sharkey & Waldron, 1990) than elsewhere, and it was destructive in both settings, breeding smoldering resentment and ill will. More rarely, people embarrassed others either to demonstrate their power over them ("I wanted to show who was boss") or simply to entertain themselves ("I wanted to see what she would do").

Audiences were not necessarily being malicious when they concocted predicaments, however; half the time they were simply trying to be *friendly*. People poked fun at others or arranged outrageous birthday surprises in order to give them a good time and show them how much they were liked. People also embarrassed others as part of an introduction or initiation into a new group of cronies. Indeed, intentional embarrassment could be a sign of solidarity, affection, and other good intentions: People were generally more likely to try to embarrass their friends and lovers than they were to embarrass strangers and mere acquaintances (Sharkey, 1993).

Thus, half of the embarrassments intentionally caused by others were meant to be friendly, and half were not. Regardless of what the audiences were trying to accomplish, however, most intentional embarrassments were negative experiences for the recipients. The targets were usually more embarrassed than the instigators of the incidents thought they were, so the episodes were usually more unpleasant than the audiences believed (Sharkey, Diggs, & Kim, 1995). Moreover, the embarrassed targets of such incidents usually considered the instigators to be more selfish than the instigators themselves thought they were being (Sharkey et al., 1995). Ordinarily, then, intentional embarrassments were more divisive than benign, and they fulfilled their objectives less often than their creators thought they did (Sharkey, 1992). If one is hoping to please a partner with a "memorable surprise" or "just good fun," intentional embarrassment appears to be a risky enterprise. Petronio et al. (1989) found that the more often relationship partners embarrassed each other, the less satisfying and the shorter their relationship tended to be. There are better ways to show affection than with embarrassment.

## RESPONSES ACROSS CULTURES

Responses to embarrassing predicaments have been studied in more than 1,300 people in six European countries (Edelmann et al., 1987; Edelmann & Neto, 1989) and Japan (Cupach & Imahori, 1993; Edelmann & Iwawaki, 1987; Imahori & Cupach, 1994; Sueda & Wiseman, 1992), and in thousands of other people in the United States. There's no question that all of the reactions I have described in both actors and observers occur around the world. Moreover, there are no meaningful differences in the relative frequencies with which the various responses are used in Greece, Italy, Portugal, Spain, Germany, and the United Kingdom, and the reactions of people in those European countries closely resemble those of people in Japan, as well (Edelmann, 1994). For the most part, there seems to be a remarkable similarity in the ways people choose to respond to embarrassment worldwide.

The few cross-cultural differences that exist seem to be linked to the distinction between individualistic and collectivistic cultures mentioned in Chapter 6. As you may recall, the United States has a society in which people celebrate their individuality and autonomy whereas Japan's culture stresses a person's interdependence with and connections to others; the two countries differ more in this respect than most other countries do. Similar events cause embarrassment in the two countries, but Japanese people may be more embarrassable on the whole (see Chapter 6), and there appear to be some differences in responses to embarrassment, too. Sueda and Wiseman (1992) asked adults in both countries how they thought they would react to various predicaments and found that U.S. respondents believed they "might use" justifications and humor in situations in which Japanese respondents thought they would "probably not use" such tactics. The U.S. sample thus liked responses that minimized the severity of a predicament more than their Japanese counterparts did. In contrast, the two groups did not differ in their expressed likelihood of using apologies, excuses, evasion, or remediation.

Sueda and Wiseman (1992) posed hypothetical situations to their respondents, however, whereas Imahori and Cupach (1994) collected accounts of actual past embarrassments from American and Japanese college students. In this sample, the Japanese reported using remediation more often than the Americans did, while the Americans reported more frequent use of humor. These differences were replicated when Cupach and Imahori (1993) focused on recalled instances of embarrassment resulting from audience provocation. In that study, Japanese students said they had tried to apologize for or remediate the situation in about a third of such events, whereas the American students reported doing so about a fifth of the time. On the other hand, the American sample reported laughing off 1 of every 8 such provocations, whereas the Japanese students responded with humor to only 1 of every 25 such events.

Thus, there is evidence that people in the United States treat embarrassing incidents lightly and humorously more often than do people in Japan. Similarly, although Edelmann and Iwawaki (1987) found scant differences in the use of humor by embarrassed actors in Japan and the United Kingdom, observers of others' embarrassments joked about them more often in the United Kingdom than in Japan. (Observers were more empathic in the United Kingdom, too.) Of course, we should not lose sight of the broader pattern that suggests that people's responses to embarrassment are remarkably similar no matter where you go. Still, the few cross-cultural differences that do exist support the possibility that embarrassment is treated a bit more seriously in collectivistic cultures (where one's transgressions ordinarily reflect more on other people) than in individualistic societies.

## SOME FINAL POINTS

The cross-cultural studies also reaffirm the conclusion that, around the world, *audiences usually respond in reassuring, supportive, or cooperative ways that help embarrassed actors regain their poise* (see Edelmann, 1994). This is an important fact that is central to an appropriate understanding of the usual functions of embarrassment in daily life. When we were children, this may not have been so; kids respond to others' embarrassments with more teasing and heckling than adults do (Stonehouse & Miller, 1994). Adults don't always help us recover from embarrassment either, and sometimes our predicaments are even caused by others. Nevertheless, it's important to realize that, as adults, witnesses to our embarrassments are more often kindly and benign than punitive and malicious.

Now, it's true that this prediction is based on general patterns that may mask certain complexities. Certainly, on average, audiences are more often kind than cruel. On the other hand, these usual responses may be based on predicaments of average severity and on normal reactions from the embarrassed actors themselves. As a person's predicament becomes severe and portrays the person more negatively, audiences should reasonably be less sympathetic and go to less trouble to help the person save face (Cupach & Metts, 1990; Schlenker, 1980). Moreover, as any substantial harm is done to them, observers are increasingly likely to be distressed and surly instead of affable and obliging. It's possible, then, that the very people who are the most embarrassed (because they deserve to be), and who would profit most from an audience's aid, are least likely to get it.

However, our own responses affect how others behave: An actor's initial response to an incident sets the scene for the audience's reply (Sharkey & Stafford, 1990). Actors who choose moderate, conciliatory responses to their embarrassments undoubtedly make it easier for their audiences to answer with empathic understanding and support. On the other hand, actors who either overreact or underreact to their predicaments are likely to be treated less tolerantly. Actors who are too intense are either likely to flee entirely, preventing the audience from helping, or stay and seem inept with emotion that appears out of proportion to the circumstances. Either way, they make an undesirable impression that may leave an audience cold (Levin & Arluke, 1982). Those who do not seem sufficiently concerned by their predicaments risk different, but also negative, evaluations from others. Moral, considerate, benevolent people are *supposed* to be embarrassed by their minor misbehaviors, and those who can blithely shrug off such actions aren't as likable as those who get appropriately upset (Semin & Manstead, 1982; Semin & Papadopoulou, 1990).

So, there are no guarantees. Audiences are not always supportive, and embarrassed people sometimes get a harsh reception. However, audiences definitely tend to be more tolerant and understanding than most of us think (Semin, 1982), and one thing we can do to facilitate their support is to expect it. If we anticipate help from others in overcoming a predicament instead of fearfully dreading their criticism, our embarrassment is likely to be moderate and appropriate instead of overblown, and that is just the kind of seemly reaction that is most likely to elicit liking and support (Castelfranchi & Poggi, 1990; Levin & Arluke, 1982). Instead of fearing embarrassment, we should *rely* on it, expecting it to be a useful mechanism that helps us and others overcome the inevitable pitfalls of interaction and social life.


## CONCLUSIONS

People exhibit a variety of responses to embarrassment, ranging from frantic escape to cool aplomb, but they are generally conciliatory and eager to please. Audiences can be caustic and jeering, and their reactions occasionally make predicaments worse. More often, however, others are empathic and supportive, and just as interested in overcoming the incident as the embarrassed person is. Moreover, this seems to be true all over the world.

Given this, I think it is profitable to respect, but not to fear, embarrassment. It simply isn't as bad, most of the time, as people usually think it will be. Moreover, exaggerated dread of embarrassment can be problematic. Not only is it needless, it can be disadvantageous, making it less likely that a person will respond with the moderate, appropriate chagrin that elicits favorable, supportive responses from observers. Thus, if you have an exaggerated fear of embarrassment, it may be worthwhile for you to overcome it. We'll consider how to proceed in the next chapter.

# CHAPTER 10

# *Overcoming Embarrassment*

~

They're out there. Those slippery steps, those bathrooms with the faulty locks, those garments with the weak seams, they're all waiting for us. So, too, are those mischievous coworkers and well-meaning friends who will do something to cause us chagrin. We will encounter an unending string of embarrassing circumstances throughout our lives, and there may come occasions when you wish that you were less susceptible, or even immune, to embarrassment. Indeed, for some of us, there may be real value in reducing our sensitivity to others' evaluations of us so that our embarrassments are more moderate and we handle predicaments more capably.

However, I urge you to question carefully any interest in overcoming embarrassment. Are you sure you want to? Remember that without embarrassment you'd not have a handy way of expressing chagrin for unwanted events that serves a useful function in daily life. As Bill Cupach (1994, p. 176) noted, the aversive nature of embarrassment reminds us of "the existence of social norms, as well as the importance of maintaining our own dignity and showing respect to others. Predicaments therefore offer a social mechanism for regulating interpersonal behavior in a civil manner." Despite the temporary discomfort it causes, embarrassment has effects that make it a desirable emotion.

Embarrassment is unquestionably a normal emotion, as well. It's not unusual to be flustered by awkward surprises in daily life; instead, it's *ab*normal to be heedless of what others may be thinking of us. For instance, according to their schoolteachers, adolescent boys who are prone to embarrassment tend to be less aggressive and delinquent *and* less anxious and withdrawn than are boys who are hard to embarrass; on the whole, those who seem to be moderately embarrassable also tend to be relatively free of psychopathology (Keltner, Moffitt, & Stouthamer-Loeber, 1995). Moreover, if embarrassment springs in part from the fundamental human need to belong (Baumeister & Leary, 1995), it would be unnatural to suppress it entirely; as Edward Gross (1994, p. 214) suggested, "being authentic and true to yourself also includes, quite often, allowing yourself to be embarrassed. To try to deny it to yourself is really denying your own humanity."

Thus, embarrassment that fits its situation is both appropriate and adaptive, and we should not wish to eradicate it completely. Instead, it seems most sensible to try to be moderately embarrassable and to experience embarrassments of medium intensity. We should strive to avoid what Peggy Thoits (1990) calls "emotional deviance," experiences of embarrassment "that differ in quality or degree from what is expected in given situations" (p. 181), and, importantly, such deviance includes embarrassments that are either too intense *or* too slight. It is normal and advantageous to experience moderate embarrassment when the situation calls for it (Levin & Arluke, 1982; Semin & Manstead, 1982), and one should seek to minimize one's susceptibility only if it is out of line.

On the other hand, there's no question that some people would be better off if they were able to face embarrassing situations with greater poise and aplomb. Chronic blushers, who frequently rearrange their lives to minimize their chances of being embarrassed by their blushing, often need such help. Their chronic dread of random embarrassment is often a central facet of their social lives, and is very disadvantageous. One of Edelmann's (1990a, p. 42) respondents reported the following:

> "I'm a 47-year-old man whose life has been ruined by blushing. My social life is very limited; I don't go anywhere. . . . Keeping a job is almost impossible because I blush even in a simple conversation. . . . You suddenly realize that you have virtually cut yourself off from people because of your blushes."

Further, as we noted in Chapter 8, the fear of embarrassment that accompanies chronic blushing is often so severe that sufferers can be properly diagnosed as suffering from social phobia. Such people are paralyzed by the thought of public scrutiny because they are terrified that they will do something embarrassing (Marshall, 1994).

This is dread of embarrassment at its worst, and because it can be so debilitating, researchers and therapists have explored a number of potential means of coping with chronic blushing. As a result, although few readers of this book will be so afflicted, chronic blushing provides a good starting point for discussion of the strategies with which embarrassment may be overcome.

## COPING WITH CHRONIC BLUSHING

Chronic blushers have been hooked to biofeedback devices that signalled them about the temperature of (Götestam, Melin, & Olsson, 1976) or the blood flow in (Rein, Giltvedt, & Götestam, 1988) their cheeks, but neither procedure helped them bring their blushing under control. In fact, this is not surprising. Because it is regulated by the autonomic nervous system, blushing is hard (if not impossible) for people to control consciously. People can neither blush on demand nor simply command themselves to stop blushing, even with good information that tells them what their cheeks are doing.

### Paradoxical Intention

However, a therapeutic approach that actually emphasizes a person's lack of control over blushing may often be of some help. Several people have been asked to *try* to blush, as often as possible, during the course of their therapy (Boeringa, 1983; Lamontagne, 1978; Timms, 1980). This approach uses the strategy of *paradoxical intention*, in which a person willfully attempts to bring on unwanted symptoms; for chronic blushing, the therapist's instructions may say, "I want you to *deliberately* practice blushing. Tell yourself to blush at all times: when you're alone, and when you're with people" (Salter, 1949, p. 106). If the person is unable to produce a blush, he or she may be told to try harder, and to keep working until he or she gets it right (Boeringa, 1983). Of course, people find that they cannot make themselves blush with any amount of practice, and, curiously, they may begin blushing less in other situations, too. In Lamontagne's (1978) case study, a young man who was suffering one long, intrusive blush per day was asked to practice blushing in various contexts for three 10-minute periods each day; months later, he was experiencing only two unwanted blushes per month.

### Cognitive Therapy

Paradoxical intention therapy can apparently be helpful, but it doesn't provide people with any insight or understanding into the origins of their problematic blushing. In particular, nobody seems to know for sure *why* paradoxical intention therapy works at all (Tennen & Affleck, 1991)! For that reason, other therapists have turned to forms of treatment that share the useful assumption that problems spring from the way people think.

Cognitive therapies all suggest that the manner in which people interpret and conceptualize important events underlies their emotional

reactions to them. "You feel the way you think," assert these practitio-
ners (A. Ellis & Harper, 1975, p. 8), and if a person's fear of embarrassment is out of control, the person must be thinking about embarrassment
in a mistaken, maladaptive way (A. T. Beck & Emery, 1985). One type
of cognitive therapy, rational–emotive therapy (RET), maintains that
people get into trouble when they hold specific wrong-headed, or
irrational, beliefs that set up exaggerated, inappropriate emotional responses. Such beliefs are usually absolutist, creating illogical standards
that are difficult (or impossible) to attain. For instance, a prime candidate for RET might have this stream of thought about blushing (see
Dryden, 1987):

> "My public behavior must be impeccable. If it is not perfect, then
> others will laugh and jeer and reject me, and will think me a complete
> fool. My blushing shows others that I am inept and unskilled. They
> will despise me, and that will be horrible. I will not be able to endure
> the humiliation the next time I blush."

You can see how someone with that outlook would be both more affected
by public scrutiny and more mortified when blushing occurs! (I hope
you can also see, having read this book, just how irrational those beliefs
are.)

People participating in RET and other cognitive therapies (e.g., J. S.
Beck, 1995) are first asked to identify their problematic beliefs. Then,
with the aid of a supportive therapist, they go about changing them,
keeping track of their old, "bad" cognitive habits and rehearsing healthier alternatives. This general strategy is often an effective treatment for
social anxiety (Glass & Shea, 1986), and can help reduce social phobia
and chronic blushing, as well (Heimberg, Liebowitz, Hope, & Schneier,
1995; Scholing & Emmelkamp, 1993). One research team paired RET
with a paradoxical intention treatment and reduced a fellow's episodes
of severe blushing from roughly one per day to one per week (Mersch,
Hildebrand, Lavy, Wessel, & van Hout, 1992). Cognitive therapy for
chronic blushing may also be particularly effective in group settings
where similar individuals can benefit from others' insights and, more
importantly, enjoy their social support (Heimberg et al., 1995).

## Other Strategies

Other strategies are also possible. One woman who had been blushing
six or seven times a day enjoyed some success through hypnosis (Welsh,
1978). When she was in a trance, the therapist induced a flush with
"warm" images such as a hot shower, and then asked her to envision

"being in a nice cool tub of water" (Welsh, p. 214); her flushes would then diminish. With repeated practice of this sort, she was able to conjure up helpful "cool" images readily, and her blushing episodes ultimately dwindled to only one per day.

An entirely different approach is systematic desensitization, which directly combats the anxious arousal chronic blushers attach to the prospect of social scrutiny. In this procedure, people are first shown how to relax and are then taught to stay calm as they gradually approach a feared situation more and more closely. Slowly but surely, they learn to face the situation with reasonable composure. By using this technique, Scholing and Emmelkamp (1993) were able to reduce the tendency of chronic blushers to avoid social situations.

If people fear embarrassment because they lack interactive skill, then specific training in social skills may also be of some use. Skills training typically involves the observation and modeling of others' effective behavior, coupled with direct instruction, role playing, and guided rehearsal of one's developing talents in real-life situations. This approach can help reduce social phobia (Wlazlo, Schroeder-Hartwig, Hand, Kaiser, & Munchau, 1990), but is probably most appropriate for a limited audience: "Most people with social phobia do not really lack basic social skills but rather are constrained from practicing them by fear, negative thoughts, and avoidance" (Marshall, 1994, p. 177).

Finally, four types of psychoactive drugs may help chronic blushers overcome the pessimistic mood and anxious arousal with which they enter social situations (Marshall, 1992, 1994). Beta-blockers such as propanolol (brand name Inderal) reduce autonomic symptoms such as sweating, tremors, and rapid pulse rate, and are usually used to treat hypertension. Benzodiazepine tranquilizers such as alprazolam (Xanax) reduce anxiety. Monoamine oxidase inhibitors such as phenelzine (Nardil) elevate mood by influencing the breakdown of certain neurotransmitters in the brain. Antidepressants such as fluoxetine (Prozac) may also be used. Each of these agents may be helpful for some sufferers, but they are not innocuous drugs and should be used under a physician's direction. They also have general effects on anxiety, mood, and arousal that are not at all specific to exaggerated fears of embarrassment.

### Eclectic Self-Help at Home

Several guided therapies can evidently be useful in treating social phobia, but many chronic blushers are no doubt interested in gaining better control of themselves on their own, without a therapist's or physician's help. For that reason, a self-directed treatment program devised by Robert Edelmann (1990a) is of particular note. Edelmann suggested that rational thinking be integrated with (1) relaxation exercises, to help people face public scrutiny with less jittery arousal; and (2) exercises to build self-confidence, to enhance people's optimism about gaining self-control. Relaxation training begins with the systematic tensing of specific muscles throughout the body that teaches a person what it feels like to be really relaxed. One is asked to tense some muscles (for instance, "make a fist, as tight as you can, and hold it for 10 seconds") and then relax, letting the muscles go loose. As this process is repeated with further regions of the body, one is also invited to take slow, deep, regular breaths and to envision a peaceful, calming scene (such as a warm sunset that leaves one more and more relaxed with each small movement of the sun toward the horizon). With practice, one can voluntarily relax at will, calming oneself when public scrutiny is imminent or even after embarrassment has already occurred.

Edelmann also encouraged people to feel better about themselves by accentuating their strengths instead of their weaknesses and by working toward effective self-control with concrete short- and long-term goals. An important aid to this process is keeping track of one's blushes and embarrassments, noting what happened, what one did and thought, and how others responded. Maintaining such records allows one to monitor desirable change, and often provides clear data showing that such incidents aren't as bad as one often fears they are.

The final component of Edelmann's program is an inventory of one's thoughts when unwanted blushes occur. He urged people to identify patterns of negative thinking that magnified the severity and importance of their blushing episodes, and to replace them with healthier cognitions that emphasized their preparedness for, and control over, social situations. Three aspects of this strategy deserve mention. First, Edelmann (1990a) encouraged people to keep optimistic thoughts, or "positive self-talk," running through their minds. When unwanted blushes intrude, he suggested thinking, "It's not the worst thing that could happen to me," or "I can handle this challenge" (p. 73). Second, Edelmann stressed the value of distracting oneself from one's blushes by redirecting one's attention to something else; instead of fretting about one's conspicuous cheeks, for instance, one could dispassionately examine some detail of someone else's appearance or behavior. (In one of my embarrassment studies, similar bland, distracting instructions to "watch for hand gestures and general shifts in [others'] body carriage" kept people from experiencing empathic embarrassment when they watched someone else perform embarrassing tasks [Miller, 1987].) Finally, borrowing a tactic from RET, Edelmann suggested that people determine whether their fears are rational with a "what-if" analysis that inspects what would happen if their fears were realized. By pondering *"what if* the worst possible thing *did* happen and you blushed" (p. 75), people can analyze the consequences of unwanted blushing in a more objective, less emotional way.

Edelmann's (1990a) self-help program thus combines elements of diverse therapies such as desensitization and cognitive therapy (e.g., A. T. Beck & Emery, 1985; Scholing & Emmelkamp, 1993), and it may be beneficial to many chronic blushers; although he reports no formal data concerning the outcomes of the program, Edelmann (1990a, p. 77) does provide many happy testimonials:

> "Once you feel more in control of your thoughts you become less concerned with what others are thinking. I have gradually felt more in control of my blushing and that things really are not so bad. As I feel more in control so my confidence is slowly but surely beginning to grow."

In any case, whether through concerted individual efforts or an organized therapy, the extreme reactions of chronic blushers appear to be amenable to change. This is good news for the rest of us, because it suggests that nearly everyone should be able to cope better with embarrassment if he or she so chooses; if people with debilitating fears of embarrassment and blushing can substantially reduce their worries, then those of us who merely wish to feel more comfortable during our ordinary embarrassments ought to be successful as well. On the other hand, as we have seen, chronic blushing and social phobia have been treated with a dizzying array of interventions variously seeking to reduce arousal, train new skills, restructure cognitions, or make blushing per se less likely. Normal people who wish to gain more control of embarrassing situations may be able to profit from several of these tactics, but they need to know where to start.

## FOCUSING ONE'S EFFORTS

Because embarrassment springs from temporary failures of impression management, a model of social distress proposed by Mark Leary and Barry Schlenker (Leary, 1987, 1995; Leary & Kowalski, 1995; Schlenker & Leary, 1982) is pertinent here. Schlenker and Leary averred that people suffer social anxiety when they are motivated to make a particular impression on others but doubt that they will be able to do so. As a result, any influence that (1) increases a person's desire to be seen in a certain way by others, or (2) decreases the person's perceived ability to make that impression, should increase the amount of concern, anxiety, or embarrassment the person experiences in that situation.

This integrative perspective has the enormous value of explaining why certain treatments for various social anxieties work better for some people than for others (Leary & Kowalski, 1995). For instance, some shy people may be anxious and inhibited because they have an excessive need for social approval and worry too much about getting strangers to like them; they may be too dependent on the good will of everyone they meet, or may take to heart the evaluations of others to whom they should be indifferent. In such cases, a cognitive therapy that helps them reduce their need for approval may be especially effective. However, other people with normal motivation may be shy because they doubt their social skills; they may correctly perceive that their skills are deficient, or they may have fine skills that they simply underestimate (Curran, Wallander, & Fischetti, 1980). Straightforward social skills training would be useful for those whose problems would be solved by the acquisition of better talents (Alden & Cappe, 1986), but it would be of little service to those who misjudge skills they already possess; in that case, cognitive therapy involving more positive self-talk and accurate self-perception would be warranted.

When it is used to conceptualize embarrassment, the Schlenker–Leary model can help us focus our efforts on the strategies for change that will do us the most good. In embarrassing predicaments, people *should* doubt their abilities to convey a desired impression because they have already failed to do so; a threat to "face" has *already occurred*, regardless of one's level of social skill. For that reason, a focus on a person's level of social skill—and, correspondingly, on the person's confidence in his or her self-presentational abilities—is usually of less value in understanding a person's embarrassment than it is in understanding other kinds of social concerns. In Chapter 6, for instance, I mentioned that chronic shyness is highly correlated with perceived deficiencies in both one's social skill and one's social self-confidence. This suggests that skill training and exercises to bolster self-esteem should be effective means of ameliorating shyness, and they are (Alden & Cappe, 1986; van der Molen, 1990). In contrast, a person's embarrassability is completely unrelated to his or her global level of social skill, and it doesn't have much to do with self-confidence (Miller, 1995b). Embarrassment begins when unwanted impressions have already been made, so neither acquiring new skills nor increasing self-confidence is likely to be of as much use in helping people master their embarrassments as are tactics that focus on people's motivation to impress others.

Those motivations are pivotal because the intensity of our embarrassments hinges on the level of our concerns for what others are thinking of us; whatever our level of social skill, if we simply did not care what others thought of us, we would not be embarrassable (Miller, 1996). Conversely, susceptibility to embarrassment increases when people want to avoid social disapproval and are motivated to convey normative, appropriate impressions. In particular, people who dread public rule violations and expect the worst when they occur may become embarrassed in ordinary situations in which unremarkable behavior is required. Thus, strategies that address the strength of people's concerns about others' judgments of them—that reduce their motivations to make particular impressions—may be especially useful in reducing the severity of the embarrassment people experience when predicaments occur.

Unfortunately, this may not be an easy task. As Leary (1995, p. 43) noted, "we find it difficult to be unconcerned with what others think even when we know it doesn't matter." However, change is possible, and modifications in people's thinking are probably more useful in this regard than are alternatives such as relaxation or desensitization (Kanter & Goldfried, 1979). As Goldfried (1979, p. 147) argued, "training in realistic thinking" is probably more efficacious than other strategies in cases in which problems are "mediated by concerns regarding the evaluations of others."

Two different types of cognitive modifications may help lower excessive concern with what others think (Leary, 1987; Leary & Kowalski, 1990). First, people can become less self-conscious (Alden & Cappe, 1986). Instead of continually focusing on others' judgments of them, people may be able to redirect their attention to other aspects of the situation. Aaron Beck and Gary Emery (1985) advocated a "decentering" technique in their cognitive therapy that encouraged people to challenge the assumption that others were always interested in, and were evaluating, them. Beck and Emery suggested that by studying others' actual behavior more closely instead of worrying about what they must be thinking, people might feel less conspicuous in social predicaments. Edelmann (1990a) included a similar focus-of-attention idea in his self-help program for chronic blushing.

However, people often *are* the legitimate centers of attention when they become embarrassed, so a second strategy of trying to reduce their fear of social disapproval may be more beneficial. Cognitive therapists Albert Ellis and Robert Harper (1975) asserted that desires for (1) unanimous acceptance and approval from others and (2) behavioral perfection were two of the most common irrational wishes that caused people trouble. Ellis and Harper (p. 198) urged people to "dispute the belief that you must feel loved or accepted by every significant person for almost everything you do . . . keep the approval of others as a *desirable* but not *necessary* goal." Further, they invited people to "give up the notion that you must act quite competently, adequately, and achievingly. Try to *do* or to do *well* rather than to do *perfectly*" (p. 198). Toward that end, Ellen Klass (1990) suggested that people critique two specific beliefs. First, she asked people to ponder dispassionately the probability of negative evaluation from others, estimating the plausible likelihood that others really would dislike them because of what they had done. Questions such as "Are they really going to hate me for tripping on that step?" and "Do *I* hate people for tripping on steps?" would be advantageous here.

Klass also encouraged people to rethink the importance of any negative evaluations that do result (e.g., "So what if they think I'm a jerk? Does it really matter?"). This "what-if" strategy was also advocated by Edelmann (1990a), and is part of A. T. Beck and Emery's (1985) "decatastrophizing" technique that asks people to contemplate the consequences they fear to make sure that they're all that frightening. In addition to thinking them over, people can also experience some potential embarrassments first hand to see just how fearsome they are. Walen, DiGiuseppe, and Dryden (1992) suggested that people break some social norms on purpose to get used to dealing with and deflecting trivial disapproval from others. (I've got one such idea for you: Try greeting and shaking hands with all the strangers who join you on an elevator. When you can do that with complete aplomb, you're becoming less embarrassable.) The final goal, according to cognitive therapists, is to feel appropriate mild regret or disappointment over flawed public performances while refraining from feeling extreme embarrassment when it is unnecessary and irrational (Dryden, 1987).

No one scheme for coping with embarrassment is likely to be the best for everyone, and multifaceted strategies that include aspects of various approaches are often the wisest choice (see Scholing & Emmelkamp, 1993, and van der Molen, 1990). However, excessive embarrassability depends more on oversensitivity to negative social evaluation than on any other contributing influence, so attempts to relax people's excessively high standards for desirable conduct and to moderate their needs for social approval are often profitable places to start.

## BEING THE MASTER OF ONE'S EMBARRASSMENTS

At last, here at the end of the book, I think it is incumbent upon me to offer you some integrative, concrete suggestions for coping with embarrassment. Let me first remind you that if you dislike embarrassment, you're not alone. All normal people are susceptible to the chagrin and flustered mortification that accompanies social predicaments, and it is an uncomfortable state. However, if you're *really* averse to embarrassment, you're probably making it out to be more fearsome and damaging than it really is. People who are particularly embarrassable probably dread the evaluations of others more than they should (Miller, 1995b); they may perceive the reactions of others toward them to be more negative than they really are (see Leary, Kowalski, & Campbell, 1988), and they probably underestimate their own abilities to deal with embarrassing predicaments (see Edelmann, 1985a). It may be reassuring to such people to learn that nobody likes being embarrassed, and everybody feels awkward and ill at ease when embarrassment strikes.

Moreover, because audiences are usually more forgiving than we tend to think they are (Metts & Cupach, 1989; Semin, 1982), we simply shouldn't worry about embarrassment as much as we sometimes do. In particular, we should be less avid about avoiding embarrassment if doing so will cause any harm to ourselves or others. Consider entertaining this rule when you ponder potential embarrassment: When a fear of embarrassment prompts you to adhere to a desirable—that is, polite or kind—social norm, follow its lead. If you feel any qualms about the prospect of being caught doing something that your parents, spouse, employer, or other significant people (including the police!) would not want you to do, let your embarrassment be your guide. On the other hand, if a fear of embarrassment is *keeping* you from doing a moral, polite, kind, or safe thing, fight back. Don't listen to your fear, and try to ignore it. Failing that, look it in the eye and question it. Use Edelmann's (1990a) tactic of "what-if" analysis to inspect your fear carefully. Of what importance is the temporary disrespect or disapproval of this particular audience compared to (1) the guilt or anger you may feel later for failing to do what you know you should have and (2) the real risks of physical or psychological harm you may run by acting in this way?

For example, as I've noted before, many people who want to engage in safe sex with a new partner may fail to do so because of the embarrassment they associate with using condoms (Hobfoll et al., 1994). They fuss about what the partner will think if they express a wish to use condoms, and fret about what the partner will think if they already have condoms on hand. They fidget about the momentary awkwardness they expect when the condom is actually donned. The result is that a condom may lie within easy reach, unused, as its owner takes a probably small, but utterly unnecessary risk. This is a case in which it might be very useful to actively combat a fear of embarrassment using a rational–emotive approach. Ask yourself: How likely is it, really, that this person will scoff at me for asking for a condom? It's entirely possible, after all, that he or she is equally interested in safe sex but just as embarrassed to bring it up. What's the worst that could happen? Is taunting or ridicule likely? If so, why would I want to share myself with such an inconsiderate, disrespectful, brusque person? (For all I know, someone who is so ill-disposed toward safe sex is more likely to be infected with something, isn't he/she?) The bottom line here, as in many cases in which a fear of embarrassment leads us astray, is that either (1) the negative consequences we dread really aren't all that likely to occur, or (2) they do occur, indicating a lack of sensitivity and polish in the audience that should lead us to care less about what they think anyway (Klass, 1990).

Sometimes there is even a third possibility, that an audience will like us *better* because we did not give in to our fear. Your lover may thank you for respecting him or her enough to want to have safe sex. In other cases, your doctor may congratulate you on your honesty, or a stranger may be grateful for your help. I have personally encountered an example of this last possibility, and it concerns another classic dilemma: What to do when someone doesn't know he has a rip in his pants. Do you tell him? If it's not too obvious and others may not notice, the best, most rational strategy may be not to mention it, particularly if it will be possible for the person to believe later that no one may have noticed. On the other hand, if it *is* obvious, and the person is participating in a social hour with dozens of other eminent colleagues and will be very abashed when he discovers the problem later, the kind thing is to tell him. The problem, of course, is that one faces a potentially awkward interaction that will be temporarily embarrassing for both parties by doing so. In my case, it was a rather famous colleague at an important professional meeting who was unaware of his disarray. He barely knew me, but I knew that he would want to know of the rip, and that I'd feel guilty for allowing a fear of trivial embarrassment to get the better of me. So, I discreetly told him. He was mildly embarrassed but grateful, and he later thanked me warmly. There's no question I did the right thing, making a new friend in the process, but I had to stifle my fear of embarrassment to do it. I learned an important lesson, too: It can be *rewarding* to master one's fear of embarrassment.

I advocate a similarly fearless, rational approach to predicaments that are unavoidable. Once you're in the grip of embarrassment, you probably won't have either the time or the resources to reflect carefully about what to do. However, you can *prepare* for future embarrassments by deciding now what you'd like to do when the time comes. This is not silly at all; you may enjoy two meaningful benefits by planning your response to your next embarrassment. First, it can be reassuring to have a tentative script for these surprising, unwanted events; they can seem less imposing when they arouse less awkward uncertainty (Klass, 1990). For example, having a script works in combating shyness: When shy college students are given explicit instructions about how to manage an upcoming meeting with a stranger, they conduct the interaction comfortably, as if they weren't shy at all (Leary, Kowalski, & Bergen, 1988). Second, there is value in mindfully committing yourself to a course of action before the need for that action arises. When people decide in advance to do something, they are much more likely to follow through and actually do it in the heat of the moment than they are if no such commitment has been made (Sherman, 1980). Thus, by planning your next response to embarrassment now, you can increase the likelihood that you will behave in a preferred way.

What responses should you choose? Let me recommend two and suggest a conditional third. First, do nothing about minor infractions. The best and simplest reaction to small miscues of various sorts is to ignore them (Gross, 1994). Sidetracking an interaction to address an unimportant goof is needless, and elaborate accounts or apologies are unwarranted. Briefly looking embarrassed is apology enough (Castelfranchi & Poggi, 1990): You'll acknowledge the incident and express your chagrin nonverbally, and nothing needs to be said. Just take a moment, collect yourself and regain your poise, and proceed as if the incident had never happened. Your audience will probably respond with evasion, too, and the event will be quickly overcome (Sharkey & Stafford, 1990).

After larger transgressions, apologize. You should also clean up your mess, if there is one, so that remediation accompanies your apology when it is appropriate. Apologies are all-purpose, conciliatory responses that are more desirable than any other verbal maneuver (Cupach et al., 1986). They make good impressions and audiences are forgiving; trust them to work.

Finally, feel free to laugh with your audience if they laugh first. If your situation amuses others, there's no need to apologize, and evasion would be awkward. Go ahead and join the fun. Above all, don't be a curmudgeon and take offense at an audience's good cheer; a wounded reaction to others' laughter would indicate that you are taking the incident (and yourself) too seriously. Others' amusement need not be belittling, as Helen Luke (1987) explains:

> We all laugh at the foibles of those around us, but those with a sense of humor do not laugh *at* a person; there is simply a feeling of delight in the ridiculous wherever it is manifest and such laughter does not condemn the other or oneself but simply enjoys the sudden recognition of the loss of proportion in all our human conflicts and contradictions. It is a healing, not a destructive thing—a delight in life, in its comedies and tragedies, its seriousness and absurdities. (p. 10)

If you embrace evasion, apologies, and humor, and eschew aggression, justifications, and flight, I think you'll be making the most reasonable choices in responding to embarrassment. Implicitly, you'll be putting embarrassing incidents into proper perspective, treating them as nuisances instead of catastrophes. Explicitly, you'll be reacting with the responses that—when they are appropriate to the situation—offer the least costly and most effective means of restoring a desired image.

The key, of course, will be having the presence of mind to implement your choices when they are needed, and that will be much easier to do if you are not overwhelmed with panicked dread of what others must be thinking of you. The intensity of your embarrassment will depend on the extent to which you fear negative evaluations from others (Miller, 1992, 1995b), and regulating that concern is another important way to master your embarrassment. Remember, audiences are usually more forgiving than we believe them to be. Even when they do make our embarrassments worse they often mean us no harm. And if they do mean you harm, consider shrugging them off and finding a new audience. None of us can please all of the people all of the time.

How should you respond when you witness others' embarrassments? I think similar reasoning applies. First, if you want to overcome the embarrassing disruption and continue the interaction, you can be guided by the initial response of the embarrassed actor. If the transgression is trivial and the actor responds with either evasion or humor, do the same. If the predicament is more severe, and particularly if any harm is done to you, expect an apology but be supportive when you get one. Accept appropriate remediation when it is offered instead of pretending that no real harm has occurred; remember that the embarrassed actor wants to restore lost "face," and remediation is a practical, realistic way to do it (Gross, 1994). On other occasions, if you want to *prolong* the actor's embarrassment for reasons of reproach or entertainment, call attention to the actor's predicament and keep teasing him or her about it; just don't expect the actor to find the episode as instructional or entertaining as you do (Sharkey et al., 1995).

All in all, don't try to become immune to embarrassment. The emotion probably evolved in our species because it was useful (Trower, Gilbert, & Sherling, 1990), and it is normal and desirable to be moderately embarrassable. Others will like you better if you become embarrassed during public predicaments than if you do not (Semin & Manstead, 1982) because your chagrin will signal appropriate concern for their opinions and seemly regret for your misbehavior (Castelfranchi & Poggi, 1990). Feel free to relax and be less frantic about what other people think of you, but don't take it too far; if you are completely unmoved by unwanted events, you may seem callous and insensitive.

Finally, when you ponder embarrassment henceforth, I hope that you'll have added respect for the emotion as a result of reading this book. It's sometimes laughable, but there are serious processes underlying embarrassment, and I think its existence speaks to important truths about humankind. We are a very social species, greatly affected by the presence and actions of our fellows, and most of us seem to perpetually monitor in some fashion what others appear to be thinking of us (Cooley, 1922/1964; Scheff, 1990). Our concerns about those judgments and our desires to maintain our inclusion in important groups are "the fuel that drives the social machine" (Scheff & Retzinger, 1991, p. 9). As a result, a lot of our behavior is motivated by a desire to avoid embarrassment and to remediate it if it occurs; arguably, "the possibility of embarrassment provides the central and continuous drama to human social life" (Schudson, 1984, p. 637). However, although it is consequential, fear of embarrassment is substantially misplaced. No one likes to feel mortified and abashed, but embarrassment usually motivates conciliatory behavior that produces desirable results, and we would all be worse off without it.

# Notes

∼

## CHAPTER 1

1. I actually did this. Most of the examples used in this book will describe real events, but the participants will generally remain anonymous.
2. This was my response. Happily, and perhaps as a result, we can laugh about it now.

## CHAPTER 2

1. The term "basic emotion" has been criticized because it implies an intensity or primacy of experience that is unwarranted (e.g., Averill, 1994). Some emotions, such as embarrassment, do seem to be particularly significant, motivating influential behavior, but "important" may be a better term (see Ekman & Davidson, 1994).

## CHAPTER 3

1. Just in case, if you're not sure, it's "Dee Flay-dur-mouse."
2. If you will permit me a personal note, I'd like to tell you about the serendipitous accident that precipitated my own scholarly interest in embarrassment. I stumbled on the notion of "empathic embarrassment" entirely by chance. When I was a graduate student, long before I read Sattler's (1965) work, I happened to watch a television broadcast of the movie *Save the Tiger*. Jack Lemmon won the Best Actor Oscar for his role in the film, playing a troubled clothing manufacturer. At one point, while addressing a large audience of buyers at his vitally important annual show, he begins to

hallucinate. He imagines his audience to be a collection of macabre skeletons wearing military helmets, and as he stands alone on the stage before the crowd, he becomes totally incapacitated; his presentation degenerates into chaos.

I sat in my bedroom, watching this invented scene on a small black-and-white TV set, and became acutely uneasy. It was difficult for me to watch. Later, curious about my reaction, I found that no one had ever empirically examined how observers react to others' social predicaments, and I set out to explore the concept I now called "empathic embarrassment." Related questions about social interaction have been of interest to me ever since, and have ultimately resulted in the creation of this book. Fortuitous accidents often play remarkable roles in our lives!

3. Evidently, my similar experience with the *Save the Tiger* film was not so unusual after all.

4. Details of these studies appear in Chapter 4.

## CHAPTER 4

1. In general, the "diary" methodology simply replicated the results of my "describe your most recent embarrassment" technique. Merely asking a large group of people to report how they were last embarrassed seems to sample various types of social predicaments reasonably well. However, two rather subtle and infrequent sources of embarrassment, "undue sensitivity" and "partner sensitivity," were identified for the first time using the diary procedure. Tracking individuals' embarrassments over time probably also provided more accurate estimates of the prevalence of these diverse predicaments. Our memories for recent embarrassments are good but not perfect, and a diary technique does seem to add some precision.

2. Each issue of YM (or *Young and Modern*) includes a page of embarrassing moments sent in by readers. People submit them voluntarily and they are screened by the editors, so they are not necessarily representative of adolescent embarrassments. Indeed, they tend to be rather single-minded, revolving around bodily functions and acceptance by peers. Nevertheless, the embarrassment devotee will find them fascinating. For unadulterated teenage agony and humiliation, it's hard to do better. This and the other accounts of embarrassment drawn from YM are copyrighted by Gruner + Jahr USA Publishing, and are reprinted with permission.

3. An event like this generated my own professional interest in embarrassment (see Chapter 3).

## CHAPTER 5

1. This idea that overwhelming changes in one's understanding of one's existence can cause psychic distress reminds me of Issac Asimov's

(1941/1990) famous short story "Nightfall." He describes a planet with six suns on which night comes, unexpectedly, only once every two-and-a-half millennia when all six stars are eclipsed at once. In the story's dramatic finish, the populace looks up into the unfamiliar night sky and realizes, for the very first time, the vastness of the cosmos and its innumerable galaxies. In their frantic effort to create light that will blot out this incomprehensible new perspective, they burn their cities to the ground. Does self-consciousness similarly defy comprehension?

2. The name is pronounced "Lar'-sun."

## CHAPTER 7

1. As a matter of fact, the single most embarrassing thing that has ever happened to me—which I am certainly not going to describe here—involved intentional behavior that did not trouble me at all until others suddenly became aware of it. My guess is that you have encountered such examples, too.

## CHAPTER 8

1. I leave to your imagination the possibilities that would result if we *could* do this.

2. The primary receptors involved here appear to be beta-adrenergic receptors controlled by norepinephrine produced by the adrenal medulla (Cutlip & Leary, 1993; Mellander et al., 1982).

## CHAPTER 9

1. We are not related. More importantly, this is the only mention of another Miller in the whole book, so, with your indulgence, I'll omit the initials (i.e., R. S. Miller) that would usually accompany the other citations of work by "Miller" elsewhere in the book.

2. Actually, there may be some people who are very hard to embarrass to whom this statement does not apply. They would be people who can brazenly, shamelessly do things that would mortify normal people, and who are thus rather immune to the dread of embarrassment that keeps the rest of us in line. They would seem to lack a conscience, which, according to H. L. Mencken (1949, p. 617), is "the inner voice that warns us that someone may be looking." In being thoroughly heedless of the evaluations of others, these people would be decidedly unusual and even *abnormal*, exhibiting all the key symptoms of an antisocial personality disorder (Kassin, 1995). This is clearly a disagreeable disorder, another indication of the desirability of a reasonable dread of embarrassment in social life.

3. The examples I will provide will imply that people want to maintain desirable, positive images for others. Although this is true for most of us most of the time, there are occasions when people want others to think badly of them (such as a gang member who wants to be feared), and such people can probably be embarrassed by, and wish to excuse, accidentally *positive* actions. Not all of us wish to be liked and accepted by others (see Leary & Miller, 1986).

4. Other authors have referred to this tactic as "avoidance," but I think "evasion" is a better term. The response does not avoid embarrassment, and should not be confused with the many things people do to prevent predicaments altogether, but it does allow one to evade most of the disruption and fluster that often accompanies an embarrassing incident. Hence, "evasion" instead of "avoidance."

5. People also just *acknowledge* their embarrassment on occasion, admitting their predicaments but otherwise offering no account. We looked for such responses—called "description" by Cupach and Metts (1990)—and were able to distinguish them reliably from full-fledged apologies (Miller et al., 1996). However, for ease of presentation, I'm treating them here as minimal (albeit vague) apologies. Such acknowledgments often concede one's responsibility ("Uh oh, I ripped my pants") and usually implicitly express the person's regret of the event ("Oh, I'm so embarrassed").

# References

⌒

Abe, K., & Masui, T. (1981). Age–sex trends of phobic and anxiety symptoms in adolescents. *British Journal of Psychiatry, 138*, 297–302.

Alden, L., & Cappe, R. (1986). Interpersonal process training for shy clients. In W. H. Jones, J. M. Cheek, & S. R. Briggs (Eds.), *Shyness: Perspectives on research and treatment* (pp. 343–355). New York: Plenum Press.

Alexander, F. (1930). *The psychoanalysis of the total personality.* New York: Nervous and Mental Disease Publishing.

American Psychiatric Association. (1994). *Diagnostic and statistical manual of mental disorders* (4th ed.). Washington, DC: Author.

Amsterdam, B. K., & Levitt, M. (1980). Consciousness of self and painful self-consciousness. *Psychoanalytic Study of the Child, 35*, 67–83.

Anderson, N. R., & Kauffman, B. E. (1991, August). *Stop kidding, I'm too embarrassed: Typical experiences of embarrassment and teasing.* Paper presented at the meeting of the American Psychological Association, San Francisco.

Anderson, N. R., & Kauffman, B. E. (1992, April). *Parents as sources of embarrassment: II. A comparison between the memories of adults and the experiences of adolescents.* Paper presented at the meeting of the Eastern Psychological Association, Boston.

Apsler, R. (1975). Effects of embarrassment on behavior toward others. *Journal of Personality and Social Psychology, 32*, 145–153.

Argyle, M., Furnham, A., & Graham, J. A. (1981). *Social situations.* Cambridge, England: Cambridge University Press.

Aronson, E., Willerman, B., & Floyd, J. (1966). The effect of a pratfall on increasing interpersonal attractiveness. *Psychonomic Science, 4*, 227–228.

Asendorpf, J. (1984). Shyness, embarrassment, and self-presentation: A control theory approach. In R. Schwarzer (Ed.), *The self in anxiety, stress, and depression* (pp. 109–114). Amsterdam: North Holland.

*205*

Asendorpf, J. (1990). The expression of shyness and embarrassment. In W. R. Crozier (Ed.), *Shyness and embarrassment: Perspectives from social psychology* (pp. 87–118). Cambridge, England: Cambridge University Press.

Asimov, I. (1990). *The complete stories* (Vol. 1). New York: Doubleday. (Original work published 1941)

Averill, J. R. (1994). In the eyes of the beholder. In P. Ekman & R. J. Davidson (Eds.), *The nature of emotion: Fundamental questions* (pp. 7–14). New York: Oxford University Press.

Babcock, M. K. (1988). Embarrassment: A window on the self. *Journal for the Theory of Social Behavior, 18,* 459–483.

Babcock, M. K., & Sabini, J. (1990). On differentiating embarrassment from shame. *European Journal of Social Psychology, 20,* 151–169.

Barry, D. (1994, April 3). Son squirms as dad hot-dogs with relish. *Texas Magazine,* p. 15.

Baumeister, R. F. (1986). *Identity: Cultural change and the struggle for self.* New York: Oxford University Press.

Baumeister, R. F. (1991). *Escaping the self: Alcoholism, spirituality, masochism, and other flights from the burden of selfhood.* New York: Basic Books.

Baumeister, R. F., & Leary, M. R. (1995). The need to belong: Desire for interpersonal attachments as a fundamental human motivation. *Psychological Bulletin, 117,* 497–529.

Baumeister, R. F., & Scher, S. J. (1988). Self-defeating behavior patterns among normal individuals: Review and analysis of common self-destructive tendencies. *Psychological Bulletin, 104,* 3–22.

Baumeister, R. F., & Tice, D. M. (1990). Anxiety and social exclusion. *Journal of Social and Clinical Psychology, 9,* 165–195.

Beck, A. T., & Emery, G. (1985). *Anxiety disorders and phobias: A cognitive perspective.* New York: Basic Books.

Beck, J. S. (1995). *Cognitive therapy: Basics and beyond.* New York: Guilford Press.

Bennett, M. (1989). Children's self-attribution of embarrassment. *British Journal of Developmental Psychology, 7,* 207–217.

Bennett, M., & Dewberry, C. (1989). Embarrassment at others' failures: A test of the Semin and Manstead model. *Journal of Social Psychology, 129,* 557–559.

Bennett, M., & Gillingham, K. (1991). The role of self-focused attention in children's attributions of social emotions to the self. *Journal of Genetic Psychology, 152,* 303–309.

Bjorklund, D. F. (1989). *Children's thinking: Developmental function and individual differences.* Pacific Grove, CA: Brooks/Cole.

Boeringa, J. A. (1983). Blushing: A modified behavioral intervention using paradoxical intention. *Psychotherapy: Theory, Research and Practice, 20,* 441–444.

Bolwig, N. (1978). Communicative signals and social behaviour of some African monkeys: A comparative study. *Primates, 19,* 61–99.

Braithwaite, D. O. (1995). Ritualized embarrassment at "coed" wedding and baby showers. *Communication Reports, 8,* 145–157.

Brody, L. R., & Hall, J. A. (1993). Gender and emotion. In M. Lewis & J. M. Haviland (Eds.), *Handbook of emotions* (pp. 447–460). New York: Guilford Press.

Brown, B. R. (1968). The effects of need to maintain face on interpersonal bargaining. *Journal of Experimental Social Psychology, 4,* 107–122.

Brown, B. R. (1970). Face-saving following experimentally induced embarrassment. *Journal of Experimental Social Psychology, 6,* 255–271.

Brown, B. R., & Garland, H. (1971). The effects of incompetency, audience acquaintanceship, and anticipated evaluative feedback on face-saving behavior. *Journal of Experimental Social Psychology, 7,* 490–502.

Browne, J. (1985). Darwin and the expression of the emotions. In D. Kohn (Ed.), *The Darwinian heritage* (pp. 307–326). Princeton, NJ: Princeton University Press.

Bruch, M. A., Giordano, S., & Pearl, L. (1986). Differences between fearful and self-conscious shy subtypes in background and current adjustment. *Journal of Research in Personality, 20,* 172–186.

Buck, R. (1991). Temperament, social skills, and the communication of emotion: A developmental–interactionist view. In D. G. Gilbert & J. J. Conley (Eds.), *Personality, social skills, and psychopathology: An individual differences approach* (pp. 85–105). New York: Plenum Press.

Buck, R. W., & Parke, R. D. (1972). Behavioral and physiological response to the presence of a friendly or neutral person in two types of stressful situations. *Journal of Personality and Social Psychology, 24,* 143–153.

Bulmer, M. (1979). Concepts in the analysis of qualitative data. *Sociological Review, 27,* 651–677.

Buss, A. H. (1980). *Self-consciousness and social anxiety.* San Francisco: Freeman.

Buss, A. H. (1986). *Social behavior and personality.* Hillsdale, NJ: Erlbaum.

Buss, A. H., Iscoe, I., & Buss, E. H. (1979). The development of embarrassment. *Journal of Psychology, 103,* 227–230.

Buss, D. M. (1990). Evolutionary social psychology: Prospects and pitfalls. *Motivation and Emotion, 14,* 265–286.

Buss, L. (1978). [Does overpraise cause embarrassment?] Unpublished raw data, University of Texas, Austin.

Cacioppo, J. T., Klein, D. J., Berntson, G. G., & Hatfield, E. (1993). The psychophysiology of emotion. In M. Lewis & J. M. Haviland (Eds.), *Handbook of emotions* (pp. 119–142). New York: Guilford Press.

Capps, L., Yirmiya, N., & Sigman, M. (1992). Understanding of simple and complex emotions in non-retarded children with autism. *Journal of Child Psychology and Psychiatry, 33,* 1169–1182.

Castelfranchi, C., & Poggi, I. (1990). Blushing as a discourse: Was Darwin wrong? In W. R. Crozier (Ed.), *Shyness and embarrassment: Perspectives from social psychology* (pp. 230–251). Cambridge, England: Cambridge University Press.

Cheek, J. M., & Briggs, S. R. (1990). Shyness as a personality trait. In W. R. Crozier (Ed.), *Shyness and embarrassment: Perspectives from social psychology* (pp. 315–337). Cambridge, England: Cambridge University Press.

Cheek, J. M., Carpentieri, A. M., Smith, T. G., Rierdan, J., & Koff, E. (1986).

Adolescent shyness. In W. Jones, J. Cheek, & S. Briggs (Eds.), *Shyness: Perspectives on research and treatment* (pp. 105–115). New York: Plenum Press.

Cheek, J. M., & Melchior, L. A. (1990). Shyness, self-esteem, and self-consciousness. In H. Leitenberg (Ed.), *Handbook of social and evaluation anxiety* (pp. 47–82). New York: Plenum Press.

Cialdini, R. B., Borden, R., Thorne, A., Walker, M., Freeman, S., & Sloane, L. T. (1976). Basking in reflected glory: Three (football) field studies. *Journal of Personality and Social Psychology, 34,* 366–375.

Clore, G. L., & Ortony, A. (1991). What more is there to emotion concepts than prototypes? *Journal of Personality and Social Psychology, 60,* 48–50.

Cody, M. J., & McLaughlin, M. L. (1985). Models for the sequential construction of accounting episodes: Situational and interactional constraints on message selection and evaluation. In R. L. Street, Jr., & J. N. Cappella (Eds.), *Sequence and pattern in communicative behavior* (pp. 50–69). Baltimore: Edward Arnold.

Cooley, C. H. (1964). *Human nature and the social order.* New York: Schocken Books. (Original work published 1922)

Coser, R. (1960). Laughter among colleagues: A study of the social functions of humor among the staff of a mental hospital. *Psychiatry, 23,* 81–95.

Crozier, W. R. (1990). Introduction. In W. R. Crozier (Ed.), *Shyness and embarrassment: Perspectives from social psychology* (pp. 1–15). Cambridge, England: Cambridge University Press.

Crozier, W. R., & Burnham, M. (1990). Age-related differences in children's understanding of shyness. *British Journal of Developmental Psychology, 8,* 179–185.

Crozier, W. R., & Russell, D. (1992). Blushing, embarrassability and self-consciousness. *British Journal of Social Psychology, 31,* 343–349.

Csikszentmihalyi, M., & Larson, R. (1984). *Being adolescent: Conflict and growth in the teenage years.* New York: Basic Books.

Cupach, W. R. (1994). Social predicaments. In W. R. Cupach & B. H. Spitzberg (Eds.), *The dark side of interpersonal communication* (pp. 159–180). Hillsdale, NJ: Erlbaum.

Cupach, W. R., & Imahori, T. T. (1993). Managing social predicaments created by others: A comparison of Japanese and American facework. *Western Journal of Communication, 57,* 431–444.

Cupach, W. R., & Metts, S. (1990). Remedial processes in embarrassing predicaments. In J. Anderson (Ed.), *Communication yearbook 13* (pp. 323–352). Newbury Park, CA: Sage.

Cupach, W. R., & Metts, S. (1992). The effects of type of predicament and embarrassability on remedial responses to embarrassing situations. *Communication Quarterly, 40,* 149–161.

Cupach, W. R., & Metts, S. (1994). *Facework.* Thousand Oaks, CA: Sage.

Cupach, W. R., Metts, S., & Hazleton, V., Jr. (1986). Coping with embarrassing predicaments: Remedial strategies and their perceived utility. *Journal of Language and Social Psychology, 5,* 181–200.

Curran, J. P., Wallander, J. L., & Fischetti, M. (1980). The importance of behavioral and cognitive factors in heterosexual–social anxiety. *Journal of Personality, 48,* 285–292.

Cutlip, W. D., II, & Leary, M. R. (1993). Anatomic and physiological bases of social blushing: Speculations from neurology and psychology. *Behavioural Neurology, 6,* 181–185.

Darvill, T. J., Johnson, R. C., & Danko, G. P. (1992). Personality correlates of public and private self-consciousness. *Personality and Individual Differences, 13,* 383–384.

Darwin, C. R. (1965). *The expression of emotions in man and animals.* Chicago: University of Chicago Press. (Original work published 1872)

Davis, J. (1981, November 26). Untitled. *Huntsville Item,* p. 6B.

Devinsky, O., Hafler, D. A., & Victor, J. (1982). Embarrassment as the aura of a complex partial seizure. *Neurology, 32,* 1284–1285.

Doherty, K., & Schlenker, B. R. (1995). Excuses as mood protection: The impact of supportive and challenging feedback from others. *Journal of Social and Clinical Psychology, 14,* 147–164.

Druian, P. R., & DePaulo, B. M. (1977). Asking a child for help. *Social Behavior and Personality, 5,* 33–39.

Drummond, P. D. (1989). Mechanism of social blushing. In N. W. Bond & D. A. T. Siddle (Eds.), *Psychobiology: Issues and applications* (pp. 363–370). Amsterdam: Elsevier Science.

Dryden, W. (1987). *Counselling individuals: The rational–emotive approach.* London: Taylor & Francis.

Eagly, A. H. (1987). *Sex differences in social behavior: A social-role interpretation.* Hillsdale, NJ: Erlbaum.

Edelmann, R. J. (1982). The effect of embarrassed reactions upon others. *Australian Journal of Psychology, 34,* 359–367.

Edelmann, R. J. (1985a). Dealing with embarrassing events: Socially anxious and non-socially anxious groups compared. *British Journal of Clinical Psychology, 24,* 281–288.

Edelmann, R. J. (1985b). Individual differences in embarrassment: Self-consciousness, self-monitoring, and embarrassability. *Personality and Individual Differences, 6,* 223–230.

Edelmann, R. J. (1987). *The psychology of embarrassment.* Chichester, England: Wiley.

Edelmann, R. J. (1990a). *Coping with blushing.* London: Sheldon Press.

Edelmann, R. J. (1990b). Embarrassment and blushing: A component-process model, some initial descriptive data and cross-cultural data. In W. R. Crozier (Ed.), *Shyness and embarrassment: Perspectives from social psychology* (pp. 205–229). Cambridge, England: Cambridge University Press.

Edelmann, R. J. (1991). Correlates of chronic blushing. *British Journal of Clinical Psychology, 30,* 177–178.

Edelmann, R. J. (1994). Embarrassment and blushing: Factors influencing face-saving strategies. In S. Ting-Toomey (Ed.), *The challenge of facework* (pp. 231–267). Albany: State University of New York Press.

Edelmann, R. J., Asendorpf, J., Contarello, A., Georgas, J., Villanueva, C., & Zammuner, V. (1987). Self-reported verbal and non-verbal strategies for coping with embarrassment in five European cultures. *Social Science Information, 26,* 869–883.

Edelmann, R. J., Asendorpf, J., Contarello, A., Zammuner, V., Georgas, J., & Villanueva, C. (1989). Self-reported expression of embarrassment in five European countries. *Journal of Cross-Cultural Psychology, 20,* 357–371.

Edelmann, R. J., & Hampson, R. J. (1979). Changes in non-verbal behaviour during embarrassment. *British Journal of Social and Clinical Psychology, 18,* 385–390.

Edelmann, R. J., & Hampson, R. J. (1981a). Embarrassment in dyadic interaction. *Social Behavior and Personality, 9,* 171–177.

Edelmann, R. J., & Hampson, R. J. (1981b). The recognition of embarrassment. *Personality and Social Psychology Bulletin, 7,* 109–116.

Edelmann, R. J., & Iwawaki, S. (1987). Self-reported expression and consequences of embarrassment in the United Kingdom and Japan. *Psychologia, 30,* 205–216.

Edelmann, R. J., & McCusker, G. (1986). Introversion, neuroticism, empathy, and embarrassibility. *Personality and Individual Differences, 7,* 133–140.

Edelmann, R. J., & Neto, F. (1989). Self-reported expression and consequences of embarrassment in Portugal and the U.K. *International Journal of Psychology, 24,* 351–366.

Edelmann, R. J., & Skov, V. (1993). Blushing propensity, social anxiety, anxiety sensitivity and awareness of bodily sensations. *Personality and Individual Differences, 14,* 495–498.

Eibl-Eibesfeldt, I. (1972). Similarities and differences between cultures in expressive movements. In R. A. Hinde (Ed.), *Nonverbal communication* (pp. 297–315). Cambridge, England: Cambridge University Press.

Eibl-Eibesfeldt, I. (1989). *Human ethology.* New York: Aldine de Gruyter.

Ekman, P. (1972). Universal and cultural differences in facial expressions of emotion. In J. K. Cole (Ed.), *Nebraska symposium on motivation, 1971* (pp. 207–283). Lincoln: University of Nebraska Press.

Ekman, P. (1992). An argument for basic emotions. *Cognition and Emotion, 6,* 169–200.

Ekman, P., & Davidson, R. J. (1993). Voluntary smiling changes regional brain activity. *Psychological Science, 4,* 342–345.

Ekman, P., & Davidson, R. J. (Eds.). (1994). *The nature of emotion: Fundamental questions.* New York: Oxford University Press.

Ekman, P., & Friesen, W. V. (1978). *Facial action coding system: A technique for the measurement of facial movement.* Palo Alto, CA: Consulting Psychologists Press.

Ellis, A., & Harper, R. A. (1975). *A new guide to rational living.* North Hollywood, CA: Wilshire.

Ellis, H. (1910). *The criminal.* New York: Charles Scribner & Sons.

Ellsworth, P. C., Friedman, H. S., Perlick, D., & Hoyt, M. E. (1978). Some effects of gaze on subjects motivated to seek or to avoid social comparison. *Journal of Experimental Social Psychology, 14,* 69–87.

English, F. (1975). Shame and social control. *Transactional Analysis Journal, 5,* 24–28.

Feinman, S., & Lewis, M. (1983). Social referencing and second order effects in ten-month-old infants. *Child Development, 54,* 878–887.

Feldman, S. (1941). On blushing. *Psychiatric Quarterly, 15,* 249–261.

Fenigstein, A., Scheier, M. F., & Buss, A. H. (1975). Public and private self-consciousness: Assessment and theory. *Journal of Consulting and Clinical Psychology, 43,* 522–527.

Ferguson, T. J., Stegge, H., & Damhuis, I. (1991). Children's understanding of guilt and shame. *Child Development, 62,* 827–839.

Fink, E. L., & Walker, B. A. (1977). Humorous responses to embarrassment. *Psychological Reports, 40,* 475–485.

Fish, B., Karabenick, S. A., & Heath, M. (1978). The effects of observation on emotional arousal and affiliation. *Journal of Experimental Social Psychology, 14,* 256–265.

Fiske, S. T. (1993). Social cognition and social perception. *Annual Review of Psychology, 44,* 155–194.

Flavell, J. H. (1993). Young children's understanding of thinking and consciousness. *Current Directions in Psychological Science, 2,* 40–43.

Flavell, J. H., Botkin, P. T., Fry, C. L., Wright, J. W., & Jarvis, P. E. (1968). *The development of role-taking and communication skills in children.* New York: Wiley.

Foss, R. D., & Crenshaw, N. C. (1978). Risk of embarrassment and helping. *Social Behavior and Personality, 6,* 243–245.

Fridlund, A. J. (1994). *Human facial expression: An evolutionary view.* San Diego: Academic Press.

Friedman, L. (1981). How affiliation affects stress in fear and anxiety situations. *Journal of Personality and Social Psychology, 40,* 1102–1117.

Frijda, N. H. (1986). *The emotions.* Cambridge, England: Cambridge University Press.

Froming, W. J., Corley, E. B., & Rinker, L. (1990). The influence of public self-consciousness and the audience's characteristics on withdrawal from embarrassing situations. *Journal of Personality, 58,* 603–622.

Fujita, F., Diener, E., & Sandvik, E. (1991). Gender differences in negative affect and well-being: The case for emotional intensity. *Journal of Personality and Social Psychology, 61,* 427–434.

Gallup, G. G., Jr. (1970). Chimpanzees: Self-recognition. *Science, 167,* 86–87.

Gallup, G. G., Jr. (1977). Self-recognition in primates: A comparative approach to the bidirectional properties of consciousness. *American Psychologist, 32,* 329–338.

Gallup, G. G., Jr. (1979). Self-recognition in chimpanzees and man: A developmental and comparative perspective. In M. Lewis & L. A. Rosenblum (Eds.), *The child and its family* (pp. 107–126). New York: Plenum Press.

Garland, H., & Brown, B. R. (1972). Face-saving as affected by subjects' sex, audiences' sex, and audience expertise. *Sociometry, 35,* 280–289.

Geen, R. G. (1991). Social motivation. *Annual Review of Psychology, 42,* 377–399.

Gibbons, F. X. (1990). The impact of focus of attention and affect on social behavior. In W. R. Crozier (Ed.), *Shyness and embarrassment: Perspectives from social psychology* (pp. 119–143). Cambridge, England: Cambridge University Press.

Glass, C. R., & Shea, C. A. (1986). Cognitive therapy for shyness and social anxiety. In W. H. Jones, J. M. Cheek, & S. R. Briggs (Eds.), *Shyness: Perspectives on research and treatment* (pp. 315–327). New York: Plenum Press.

Goffman, E. (1955). On facework: An analysis of ritual elements in social interaction. *Psychiatry, 18*, 213–231.

Goffman, E. (1956). Embarrassment and social organization. *American Journal of Sociology, 62*, 264–271.

Goffman, E. (1959). *The presentation of self in everyday life*. Garden City, NY: Doubleday.

Goldfried, M. R. (1979). Anxiety reduction through cognitive-behavioral intervention. In P. C. Kendall & S. D. Hollon (Eds.), *Cognitive-behavioral interventions: Theory, research, and procedures* (pp. 117–152). New York: Academic Press.

Gonzales, M. H. (1992). A thousand pardons: The effectiveness of verbal remedial tactics during account episodes. *Journal of Language and Social Psychology, 11*, 133–151.

Gonzales, M. H., Pederson, J. H., Manning, D. J., & Wetter, D. W. (1990). Pardon my gaffe: Effects of sex, status, and consequence severity on accounts. *Journal of Personality and Social Psychology, 58*, 610–621.

Goodall, J. (1988). *In the shadow of man* (Rev. ed.). Boston: Houghton Mifflin.

Götestam, K. G., Melin, L., & Olsson, B. (1976). Treatment of erythrophobia by cooling and temperature feedback. *Scandinavian Journal of Behavior Therapy, 5*, 153–159.

Gould, R., & Sigall, H. (1977). The effects of empathy and outcome on attribution: An examination of the divergent-perspectives hypothesis. *Journal of Experimental Social Psychology, 13*, 480–491.

Grasmick, H. G., Bursik, R. J., Jr., & Kinsey, K. A. (1991). Shame and embarrassment as deterrents to noncompliance with the law: The case of an antilittering campaign. *Environment and Behavior, 23*, 233–251.

Griffin, S. (1995). A cognitive-developmental analysis of pride, shame, and embarrassment in middle childhood. In J. P. Tangney & K. W. Fischer (Eds.), *Self-conscious emotions: The psychology of shame, guilt, embarrassment, and pride* (pp. 219–236). New York: Guilford Press.

Gross, E. (1994). *Embarrassment in everyday life: What to do about it!* Palm Springs, CA: ETC.

Gross, E., & Stone, G. P. (1964). Embarrassment and the analysis of role requirements. *American Journal of Sociology, 70*, 1–15.

Grossman, M., & Wood, W. (1993). Sex differences in intensity of emotional experience: A social role interpretation. *Journal of Personality and Social Psychology, 65*, 1010–1022.

Halberstadt, A. G., & Green, L. R. (1993). Social attention and placation theories of blushing. *Motivation and Emotion, 17*, 53–64.

Hall, J. A. (1984). *Nonverbal sex differences: Communication accuracy and expressive style*. Baltimore: Johns Hopkins University Press.

Harré, R. (1990). Embarrassment: A conceptual analysis. In W. R. Crozier (Ed.), *Shyness and embarrassment: Perspectives from social psychology* (pp. 181–204). Cambridge, England: Cambridge University Press.

Harré, R. (1995, June). *Acting from a position: Personal relations as aspects of complex discursive networks.* Paper presented at the meeting of the International Network on Personal Relationships, Williamsburg, VA.

Harré, R., & Parrott, W. G. (Eds.). (1996). *The emotions: Social, clinical, and physical dimensions of the emotions.* London: Sage.

Harris, P. L. (1993). Understanding emotion. In M. Lewis & J. M. Haviland (Eds.), *Handbook of emotions* (pp. 237–246). New York: Guilford Press.

Harris, P. R. (1990). Shyness and embarrassment in psychological theory and ordinary language. In W. R. Crozier (Ed.), *Shyness and embarrassment: Perspectives from social psychology* (pp. 59–86). Cambridge, England: Cambridge University Press.

Harter, S., & Whitesell, N. R. (1989). Developmental changes in children's understanding of single, multiple, and blended emotion concepts. In C. Saarni & P. L. Harris (Eds.), *Children's understanding of emotion* (pp. 81–116). Cambridge, England: Cambridge University Press.

Hashimoto, E., & Shimizu, T. (1988). A cross-cultural study of the emotion of shame/embarrassment: Iranian and Japanese children. *Psychologia, 31,* 1–6.

Hatfield, E., Cacioppo, J. T., & Rapson, R. L. (1993). *Emotional contagion.* Cambridge, England: Cambridge University Press.

Hatfield, E., & Rapson, R. L. (1990). Passionate love in intimate relationships. In B. Moore & A. Isen (Eds.), *Affect and social behavior* (pp. 126–151). Cambridge, England: Cambridge University Press.

Heath, C. (1988). Embarrassment and interactional organization. In P. Drew & A. Wootton (Eds.), *Erving Goffman: Exploring the interaction order* (pp. 136–160). Boston: Northeastern University Press.

Heimberg, R. G., Liebowitz, M. R., Hope, D. A., & Schneier, F. R. (Eds.). (1995). *Social phobia: Diagnosis, assessment, and treatment.* New York: Guilford Press.

Heimlich, H. J., & Uhley, M. H. (1979). The Heimlich Maneuver. *Clinical Symposia, 31,* 1–32.

Helmreich, R., Aronson, E., & LeFan, J. (1970). To err is humanizing—sometimes: Effects of self-esteem, competence, and a pratfall on interpersonal attraction. *Journal of Personality and Social Psychology, 16,* 259–264.

Helwig-Larsen, M., & Collins, B. E. (1994). The UCLA Multidimensional Condom Attitudes Scale: Documenting the complex determinants of condom use in college students. *Health Psychology, 13,* 224–237.

Herold, E. S. (1981). Contraceptive embarrassment and contraceptive behavior among young single women. *Journal of Youth and Adolescence, 10,* 233–242.

Higgins, E. T. (1989). Self-discrepancy theory: What patterns of self-beliefs cause people to suffer? In L. Berkowitz (Ed.), *Advances in experimental social psychology* (Vol. 22, pp. 93–136). New York: Academic Press.

Hobfoll, S. E., Jackson, A. P., Lavin, J., Britton, P. J., & Shperd, J. B. (1994). Women's barriers to safer sex. *Psychology and Health, 9,* 233–252.

Hochschild, A. P. (1979). Emotion work, feeling rules, and social structure. *American Journal of Sociology, 85,* 551–575.

Horowitz, E. (1962). Reported embarrassment memories of elementary school, high school, and college students. *Journal of Social Psychology, 56,* 317–325.

Imahori, T. T., & Cupach, W. R. (1994). A cross-cultural comparison of the interpretation and management of face: U.S. American and Japanese responses to embarrassing predicaments. *International Journal of Intercultural Relations, 18,* 193–219.

Izard, C. E. (1971). *The face of emotion.* New York: Appleton-Century-Crofts.

Izard, C. E. (1977). *Human emotions.* New York: Plenum Press.

Izard, C. E. (1993). Organizational and motivational functions of discrete emotions. In M. Lewis & J. M. Haviland (Eds.), *Handbook of emotions* (pp. 631–641). New York: Guilford Press.

Jellison, J. M., & Gentry, K. W. (1978). A self-presentation interpretation of the seeking of social approval. *Personality and Social Psychology Bulletin, 4,* 227–230.

Kagan, J., & Reznick, J. S. (1986). Shyness and temperament. In W. H. Jones, J. M. Cheek, & S. R. Briggs (Eds.), *Shyness: Perspectives on research and treatment* (pp. 81–90). New York: Plenum Press.

Kagan, J., Snidman, N., & Arcus, D. M. (1992). Initial reactions to unfamiliarity. *Current Directions in Psychological Science, 1,* 171–174.

Kanter, N. J., & Goldfried, M. R. (1979). Relative effectiveness of rational restructuring and self-control desensitization in the reduction of interpersonal anxiety. *Behavior Therapy, 10,* 472–490.

Karch, F. E. (1971). Blushing. *Psychoanalytic Review, 58,* 37–50.

Kassin, S. (1995). *Psychology.* Boston: Houghton Mifflin.

Kauffman, B. E., & Anderson, N. R. (1992, June). *How do you embarrass me? Let's factor analyze the ways: Self vs. parents as causes of embarrassment and teasing.* Paper presented at the meeting of the American Psychological Society, San Diego.

Kaufman, G. (1989). *The psychology of shame: Theory and treatment of shame-based syndromes.* New York: Springer.

Kelly, K. M. (1994, November). *The structure and personality correlates of the Embarrassability Scale.* Poster session presented at the meeting of the Society of Southeastern Social Psychologists, Winston-Salem, NC.

Keltner, D. (1995). Signs of appeasement: Evidence for the distinct displays of embarrassment, amusement, and shame. *Journal of Personality and Social Psychology, 68,* 441–454.

Keltner, D., & Buswell, B. N. (1996). Evidence for the distinctness of embarrassment, shame, and guilt: A study of recalled antecedents and facial expressions of emotion. *Cognition and Emotion, 10,* 155–171.

Keltner, D., Moffitt, T. E., & Stouthamer-Loeber, M. (1995). Facial expressions of emotion and psychopathology in adolescent boys. *Journal of Abnormal Psychology, 104,* 644–652.

Kemper, T. D. (1993). Sociological models in the explanation of emotions. In M. Lewis & J. M. Haviland (Eds.), *Handbook of emotions* (pp. 41–51). New York: Guilford Press.

Klass, E. T. (1990). Guilt, shame, and embarrassment: Cognitive-behavioral approaches. In H. Leitenberg (Ed.), *Handbook of social and evaluative anxiety* (pp. 385–414). New York: Plenum Press.

Kopp, C. B. (1982). The antecedents of self-regulation: A developmental perspective. *Developmental Psychology, 18,* 199–214.

Kowalski, R. M., & Brown, K. J. (1994). Psychosocial barriers to cervical cancer screening: Concerns with self-presentation and social evaluation. *Journal of Applied Social Psychology, 24,* 941–958.

LaFrance, M., & Banaji, M. (1992). Toward a reconsideration of the gender–emotion relationship. In M. S. Clark (Ed.), *Review of personality and social psychology* (pp. 178–201). Newbury Park, CA: Sage.

Lamontagne, Y. (1978). Treatment of erythrophobia by paradoxical intention. *Journal of Nervous and Mental Disease, 166,* 304–306.

Landers, A. (1994, May 1). Condom buyer not so lucky. *Houston Chronicle,* p. 7G.

Latané, B. (1981). The psychology of social impact. *American Psychologist, 36,* 343–356.

Latané, B., & Darley, J. (1970). *The unresponsive bystander: Why doesn't he help?* New York: Appleton-Century-Crofts.

Latané, B., & Harkins, S. (1976). Cross-modality matches suggest anticipated stage fright a multiplicative power function of audience size and status. *Perception and Psychophysics, 20,* 482–488.

Lazarus, R. S. (1991). *Emotion and adaptation.* New York: Oxford University Press.

Leary, M. R. (1983). A brief version of the Fear of Negative Evaluation Scale. *Personality and Social Psychology Bulletin, 9,* 371–375.

Leary, M. R. (1987). A self-presentational model for the treatment of social anxieties. In J. E. Maddux, C. D. Stoltenberg, & R. Rosenwein (Eds.), *Social processes in clinical and counseling psychology* (pp. 126–138). New York: Springer-Verlag.

Leary, M. R. (1990). Responses to social exclusion: Social anxiety, jealousy, loneliness, depression, and low self-esteem. *Journal of Social and Clinical Psychology, 9,* 221–229.

Leary, M. R. (1991). Social anxiety, shyness, and related constructs. In J. Robinson, P. Shaver, & L. Wrightsman (Eds.), *Measures of personality and social psychological attitudes* (pp. 161–194). New York: Academic Press.

Leary, M. R. (1995). *Self-presentation: Impression management and interpersonal behavior.* Madison, WI: Brown & Benchmark.

Leary, M. R., Britt, T. W., Cutlip, W. D., II, & Templeton, J. L. (1992). Social blushing. *Psychological Bulletin, 112,* 446–460.

Leary, M. R., & Dobbins, S. E. (1983). Social anxiety, sexual behavior, and contraceptive use. *Journal of Personality and Social Psychology, 45,* 1347–1354.

Leary, M. R., & Downs, D. L. (1995). Interpersonal functions of the self-esteem motive: The self-esteem system as a sociometer. In M. H. Kernis (Ed.), *Efficacy, agency, and self-esteem* (pp. 123–144). New York: Plenum Press.

Leary, M. R., & Kowalski, R. M. (1990). Impression management: A literature review and two-component model. *Psychological Bulletin, 107,* 34–47.

Leary, M. R., & Kowalski, R. M. (1995). *Social anxiety.* New York: Guilford Press.

Leary, M. R., Kowalski, R. M., & Bergen, D. J. (1988). Interpersonal information acquisition and confidence in first encounters. *Personality and Social Psychology Bulletin, 14,* 68–77.

Leary, M. R., Kowalski, R. M., & Campbell, C. D. (1988). Self-presentational concerns and social anxiety: The role of generalized impression expectancies. *Journal of Research in Personality, 22,* 308–321.

Leary, M. R., Landel, J. L., & Patton, K. M. (in press). The motivated expression of embarrassment following a self-presentational predicament. *Journal of Personality.*

Leary, M. R., & Meadows, S. (1991). Predictors, elicitors, and concomitants of social blushing. *Journal of Personality and Social Psychology, 60,* 254–262.

Leary, M. R., & Miller, R. S. (1986). *Social psychology and dysfunctional behavior: Origins, diagnosis, and treatment.* New York: Springer-Verlag.

Leary, M. R., Nezlek, J. B., Downs, D., Radford-Davenport, J., Martin, J., & McMullen, A. (1994). Self-presentation in everyday interactions: Effects of target familiarity and gender composition. *Journal of Personality and Social Psychology, 67,* 664–673.

Leary, M. R., Rejeski, W. J., Britt, T., & Smith, G. E. (1994). *Physiological differences between embarrassment and social anxiety.* Unpublished manuscript, Wake Forest University, Winston-Salem, NC.

Leary, M. R., Schreindorfer, L. S., & Haupt, A. L. (1995). The role of low self-esteem in emotional and behavioral problems: Why is low self-esteem dysfunctional? *Journal of Social and Clinical Psychology, 14,* 297–314.

Leary, M. R., Tambor, E. S., Terdal, S. K., & Downs, D. L. (1995). Self-esteem as an interpersonal monitor: The sociometer hypothesis. *Journal of Personality and Social Psychology, 68,* 518–530.

Leary, M. R., Tchividjian, L. R., & Kraxberger, B. E. (1994). Self-presentation can be hazardous to your health: Impression management and health risk. *Health Psychology, 13,* 461–470.

LeDoux, J. E. (1995). Emotion: Clues from the brain. *Annual Review of Psychology, 46,* 209–235.

Leith, K. P., & Baumeister, R. F. (in press). Why do bad moods increase self-defeating behavior? Emotion, risk-taking, and self-regulation. *Journal of Personality and Social Psychology.*

Lerman, C., Rimer, B., Trock, B., Balshem, A., & Engstrom, P. F. (1990). Factors associated with repeat adherence to breast cancer screening. *Preventive Medicine, 19,* 279–290.

Levenson, R. W. (1992). Autonomic nervous system differences among emotions. *Psychological Science, 3,* 23–27.

Levin, J., & Arluke, A. (1982). Embarrassment and helping behavior. *Psychological Reports, 51,* 999–1002.

Lewis, M. (1992). *Shame: The exposed self.* New York: Free Press.

Lewis, M. (1993). The emergence of human emotions. In M. Lewis & J. M. Haviland (Eds.), *Handbook of emotions* (pp. 223–235). New York: Guilford Press.

Lewis, M. (1995). Embarrassment: The emotion of self-exposure and evaluation. In J. P. Tangney & K. W. Fischer (Eds.), *Self-conscious emotions: The psychology of shame, guilt, embarrassment, and pride* (pp. 198–218). New York: Guilford Press.

Lewis, M., & Brooks-Gunn, J. (1979). *Social cognition and the acquisition of self.* New York: Plenum Press.

Lewis, M., & Saarni, C. (1985). Culture and emotions. In M. Lewis & C. Saarni (Eds.), *The socialization of emotion* (pp. 1–17). New York: Plenum Press.

Lewis, M., Stanger, C., Sullivan, M. W., & Barone, P. (1991). Changes in embarrassment as a function of age, sex and situation. *British Journal of Developmental Psychology, 9,* 485–492.

Lewis, M., Sullivan, M. W., Stanger, C., & Weiss, M. (1989). Self development and self-conscious emotions. *Child Development, 60,* 146–156.

Lewittes, D. J., & Simmons, W. I. (1975). Impression management of sexually motivated behavior. *Journal of Social Psychology, 96,* 39–44.

Linton, M. (1982). Transformations of memory in everyday life. In U. Neisser (Ed.), *Memory observed: Remembering in natural contexts* (pp. 77–91). San Francisco: Freeman.

Luke, H. M. (1987). The laughter at the heart of things. *Parabola, 12,* 6–17.

Maccoby, E. (1990). Gender and relationships: A developmental account. *American Psychologist, 45,* 513–520.

Maccoby, E., & Martin, J. A. (1983). Socialization in the context of the family: Parent–child interaction. In E. M. Hetherington (Ed.), *Handbook of child psychology: Vol. 4. Socialization, personality, and child development* (4th ed., pp. 1–101). New York: Wiley.

MacDonald, L. M., & Davies, M. F. (1983). Effects of being observed by a friend or stranger on felt embarrassment and attributions of embarrassment. *Journal of Psychology, 113,* 171–174.

Mackie, D. M., & Worth, L. T. (1989). Processing deficits and the mediation of positive affect in persuasion. *Journal of Personality and Social Psychology, 57,* 27–40.

Manstead, A. S. R., & Semin, G. R. (1981). Social transgressions, social perspectives, and social emotionality. *Motivation and Emotion, 5,* 249–261.

Manstead, A. S. R., & Tetlock, P. E. (1989). Cognitive appraisals and emotional experience: Further evidence. *Cognition and Emotion, 3,* 225–240.

Marcus, D. K., Wilson, J. R., & Miller, R. S. (in press). Are perceptions of emotion in the eye of the beholder? A social relations analysis of judgments of embarrassment. *Personality and Social Psychology Bulletin.*

Markus, H. R., & Kitayama, S. (1991). Culture and the self: Implications for cognition, emotion, and motivation. *Psychological Review, 98,* 224–253.

Marshall, J. R. (1992). The psychopharmacology of social phobia. *Bulletin of the Menninger Clinic, 56,* 42–49.

Marshall, J. R. (1994). *Social phobia: From shyness to stage fright.* New York: BasicBooks.

Martin, W. B. W. (1987). Students' perceptions of causes and consequences of embarrassment in the school. *Canadian Journal of Education, 12,* 277–293.

Matsumoto, D., Kudoh, T., Scherer, K., & Wallbott, H. (1988). Antecedents of and reactions to emotions in the United States and Japan. *Journal of Cross-Cultural Psychology, 19,* 267–286.

McDonald, J., & McKelvie, S. J. (1992). Playing it safe: Helping rates for a dropped mitten and a box of condoms. *Psychological Reports, 71,* 113–114.

Mellander, S., Andersson, P., Afzelius, L., & Hellstrand, P. (1982). Neural beta-adrenergic dilatation of the facial vein in man: Possible mechanism in emotional blushing. *Acta Physiologica Scandinavica, 114,* 393–399.

Mencken, H. L. (1949). *A Mencken chrestomathy.* New York: Knopf.

Mersch, P. P. A., Hildebrand, M., Lavy, E. H., Wessel, I., & van Hout, W. J. P. J. (1992). Somatic symptoms in social phobia: A treatment method based on rational emotive therapy and paradoxical interventions. *Journal of Behavior Therapy and Experimental Psychiatry, 23,* 199–211.

Mesquita, B., & Frijda, N. H. (1992). Cultural variations in emotions: A review. *Psychological Bulletin, 112,* 179–204.

Metts, S., & Bowers, J. W. (1994). Emotion in interpersonal communication. In M. L. Knapp & G. R. Miller (Eds.), *Handbook of interpersonal communication* (2nd ed., pp. 508–541). Thousand Oaks, CA: Sage.

Metts, S., & Cupach, W. R. (1989). Situational influence on the use of remedial strategies in embarrassing predicaments. *Communication Monographs, 56,* 151–162.

Miller, D. T., & Prentice, D. A. (1994). Collective errors and errors about the collective. *Personality and Social Bulletin, 20,* 541–550.

Miller, R. S. (1986). Embarrassment: Causes and consequences. In W. H. Jones, J. M. Cheek, & S. R. Briggs (Eds.), *Shyness: Perspectives on research and treatment* (pp. 295–311). New York: Plenum Press.

Miller, R. S. (1987). Empathic embarrassment: Situational and personal determinants of reactions to the embarrassment of another. *Journal of Personality and Social Psychology, 53,* 1061–1069.

Miller, R. S. (1988, August). *Embarrassability and reactions to the threat of embarrassment.* Paper presented at the meeting of the American Psychological Association, Atlanta.

Miller, R. S. (1992). The nature and severity of self-reported embarrassing circumstances. *Personality and Social Psychology Bulletin, 18,* 190–198.

Miller, R. S. (1995a). Embarrassment and social behavior. In J. P. Tangney & K. W. Fischer (Eds.), *Self-conscious emotions: The psychology of shame, guilt, embarrassment, and pride* (pp. 322–339). New York: Guilford Press.

Miller, R. S. (1995b). On the nature of embarrassability: Shyness, social evaluation, and social skill. *Journal of Personality, 63,* 315–339.

Miller, R. S. (1996). *On the social origins of a self-conscious emotion: Delineating the causes of embarrassment.* Manuscript submitted for publication.

Miller, R. S., Bowersox, K. A., Cook, R. E., & Kahikina, C. S. (1996, April). *Responses to embarrassment.* Paper presented at the meeting of the Southwestern Psychological Association, Houston.

Miller, R. S., & Fahey, D. E. (1991, August). *Blushing as an appeasement gesture: Felt, displayed, and observed embarrassment.* Paper presented at the meeting of the American Psychological Association, San Francisco.

Miller, R. S., & Leary, M. R. (1992). Social sources and interactive functions of emotion: The case of embarrassment. In M. S. Clark (Ed.), *Review of personality and social psychology* (Vol. 14, pp. 202–221). Newbury Park, CA: Sage.

Miller, R. S., & Tangney, J. P. (1994). Differentiating embarrassment and shame. *Journal of Social and Clinical Psychology, 13,* 273–287.

Modigliani, A. (1968). Embarrassment and embarrassability. *Sociometry, 31,* 313–326.

Modigliani, A. (1971). Embarrassment, facework, and eye contact: Testing a theory of embarrassment. *Journal of Personality and Social Psychology, 17,* 15–24.

Morley, R. (1983). *Pardon me, but you're eating my doily.* New York: St. Martin's Press.

Mosher, D. L., & White, B. R. (1981). On differentiating shame and shyness. *Motivation and Emotion, 5,* 61–74.

Nathanson, D. L. (1987). A timetable for shame. In D. L. Nathanson (Ed.), *The many faces of shame* (pp. 1–63). New York: Guilford Press.

Nightmare of the month. (1992, November). YM, p. 14.

Oatley, K., & Jenkins, J. M. (1992). Human emotions: Function and dysfunction. *Annual Review of Psychology, 43,* 55–85.

Ortony, A., Clore, G. L., & Collins, A. (1988). *The cognitive structure of emotions.* Cambridge, England: Cambridge University Press.

Parrott, W. G., & Harré, R. (1991). Smedslundian suburbs in the city of language: The case of embarrassment. *Psychological Inquiry, 2,* 358–361.

Parrott, W. G., Sabini, J., & Silver, M. (1988). The roles of self-esteem and social interaction in embarrassment. *Personality and Social Psychology Bulletin, 14,* 191–202.

Parrott, W. G., & Smith, S. F. (1991). Embarrassment: Actual vs. typical cases, classical vs. prototypical representations. *Cognition and Emotion, 5,* 467–488.

Pedersen, D. M., Keithly, S., & Brady, K. (1986). Effects of an observer on conformity to handwashing norm. *Perceptual and Motor Skills, 62,* 169–170.

Pennebaker, J. W., & Roberts, T. (1992). Toward a his and hers theory of emotion: Gender differences in visceral perception. *Journal of Social and Clinical Psychology, 11,* 199–212.

Petras, R., & Petras, K. (1993). *The 776 stupidest things ever said.* New York: Doubleday.

Petronio, S. (1984). Communication strategies to reduce embarrassment: Differences between men and women. *Western Journal of Speech Communication, 48,* 28–38.

Petronio, S., Olson, C., & Dollar, N. (1989). Privacy issues in relational embarrassment: Impact on relational quality and communication satisfaction. *Communication Research Reports, 6,* 21–27.

Piaget, J., & Inhelder, B. (1967). *The child's conception of space.* New York: Norton.

Pliner, P., & Chaiken, S. (1990). Eating, social motives, and self-presentation in men and women. *Journal of Experimental Social Psychology, 26,* 240–254.

Plomin, R., & Daniels, D. (1986). Genetics and shyness. In W. H. Jones, J. M. Cheek, & S. R. Briggs (Eds.), *Shyness: Perspectives on research and treatment* (pp. 63–80). New York: Plenum Press.

Plutchik, R. (1980). *Emotion: A psychoevolutionary synthesis.* New York: Harper & Row.

Rein, J. G., Giltvedt, J., & Götestam, K. G. (1988). Vasomotor feedback in the treatment of erythrophobia: An experimental case study. *European Journal of Psychiatry, 2,* 6–9.

Riggio, R. E. (1986). Assessment of basic social skills. *Journal of Personality and Social Psychology, 51,* 649–660.

Riordan, C. A., Marlin, N. A., & Kellogg, R. T. (1983). The effectiveness of accounts following transgressions. *Social Psychology Quarterly, 46,* 213–219.

Roseman, I. J., Wiest, C., & Swartz, T. S. (1994). Phenomenology, behaviors, and goals differentiate discrete emotions. *Journal of Personality and Social Psychology, 67,* 206–221.

Ruble, T. L. (1983). Sex stereotypes: Issues of change in the 1970s. *Sex Roles, 9,* 397–402.

Russell, J. A. (1991). In defense of a prototype approach to emotion concepts. *Journal of Personality and Social Psychology, 60,* 37–47.

Russell, J. A., & Fehr, B. (1994). Fuzzy concepts in a fuzzy hierarchy: Varieties of anger. *Journal of Personality and Social Psychology, 67,* 186–205.

Saarni, C. (1985). Indirect processes in affect socialization. In M. Lewis & C. Saarni (Eds.), *The socialization of emotion* (pp. 187–209). New York: Plenum Press.

Saarni, C. (1993). Socialization of emotion. In M. Lewis & J. M. Haviland (Eds.), *Handbook of emotions* (pp. 435–446). New York: Guilford Press.

Saarni, C., & Harris, P. L. (Eds.). (1989). *Children's understanding of emotion.* Cambridge, England: Cambridge University Press.

Salter, A. (1949). *Conditioned reflex therapy.* New York: Creative Age Press.

Sartre, J. P. (1956). *Being and nothingness.* New York: Citadel Press.

Sattler, J. M. (1963). The relative meaning of embarrassment. *Psychological Reports, 12,* 263–269.

Sattler, J. M. (1965). A theoretical, developmental, and clinical investigation of embarrassment. *Genetic Psychology Monographs, 71,* 19–59.

Say anything. (1991, December/1992, January). YM, p. 12.

Say anything. (1992, April). YM, p. 16.

Say anything. (1993, May). YM, p. 14.

Scheff, T. J. (1990). Socialization of emotions: Pride and shame as causal agents. In T. D. Kemper (Ed.), *Research agendas in the sociology of emotion* (pp. 291–304). Albany: State University of New York Press.

Scheff, T. J., & Retzinger, S. M. (1991). *Emotions and violence: Shame and rage in destructive conflicts.* Lexington, MA: Lexington Books.

Scherer, K. R., & Wallbott, H. G. (1994). Evidence for universality and cultural variation of differential emotion response patterning. *Journal of Personality and Social Psychology, 66*, 310–328.

Schlenker, B. R. (1980). *Impression management: The self-concept, social identity, and interpersonal relations*. Monterey, CA: Brooks/Cole.

Schlenker, B. R., & Darby, B. W. (1981). The use of apologies in social predicaments. *Social Psychology Quarterly, 44*, 271–278.

Schlenker, B. R., & Leary, M. R. (1982). Social anxiety and self-presentation: A conceptualization and model. *Psychological Bulletin, 92*, 641–669.

Schlenker, B. R., & Weigold, M. F. (1992). Interpersonal processes involving impression regulation and management. *Annual Review of Psychology, 43*, 133–168.

Scholing, A., & Emmelkamp, P. M. (1993). Cognitive and behavioural treatments of fear of blushing, sweating or trembling. *Behaviour Research and Therapy, 31*, 155–170.

Schönbach, P. (1990). *Account episodes: The management or escalation of conflict*. Cambridge, England: Cambridge University Press.

Schudson, M. (1984). Embarrassment and Erving Goffman's idea of human nature. *Theory and Society, 13*, 633–648.

Scott, J. (1989, March 1). Nancy. *Huntsville Item*, p. B6.

Scott, M. B., & Lyman, S. M. (1968). Accounts. *American Sociological Review, 33*, 46–62.

Seidner, L. B., Stipek, D. J., & Feshbach, N. D. (1988). A developmental analysis of elementary school-aged children's concepts of pride and embarrassment. *Child Development, 59*, 367–377.

Selman, R. L. (1976). Social-cognitive understanding: A guide to educational and clinical practice. In T. Lickona (Ed.), *Moral development and behavior* (pp. 299–316). New York: Holt, Rinehart & Winston.

Semin, G. R. (1982). The transparency of the sinner. *European Journal of Social Psychology, 12*, 173–180.

Semin, G. R., & Manstead, A. S. R. (1981). The beholder beheld: A study of social emotionality. *European Journal of Social Psychology, 11*, 253–265.

Semin, G. R., & Manstead, A. S. R. (1982). The social implications of embarrassment displays and restitution behavior. *European Journal of Social Psychology, 12*, 367–377.

Semin, G. R., & Papadopoulou, K. (1990). The acquisition of reflexive social emotions: The transmission and reproduction of social control through joint action. In G. Duveen & B. Lloyd (Eds.), *Social representations and the development of knowledge* (pp. 107–125). Cambridge, England: Cambridge University Press.

Seta, C. E., & Seta, J. J. (1992). Increments and decrements in mean arterial pressure as a function of audience composition: An averaging and summation analysis. *Personality and Social Bulletin, 18*, 173–181.

Shahidi, S., & Baluch, B. (1991). False heart-rate feedback, social anxiety and self-attribution of embarrassment. *Psychological Reports, 69*, 1024–1026.

Sharkey, W. F. (1991). Intentional embarrassment: Goals, tactics, and consequences. In W. R. Cupach & S. Metts (Eds.), *Advances in interpersonal communication research—1991* (pp. 105–128). Normal, IL: Personal Relationships Interest Group.

Sharkey, W. F. (1992). Uses of and responses to intentional embarrassment. *Communication Studies, 43,* 257–275.

Sharkey, W. F. (1993). Who embarrasses whom? Relational and sex differences in the use of intentional embarrassment. In P. J. Kalbfleisch (Ed.), *Interpersonal communication: Evolving interpersonal relationships* (pp. 147–168). Hillsdale, NJ: Erlbaum.

Sharkey, W. F., Diggs, R., & Kim, M. (1995). *Intentional embarrassment: Embarrassors and embarrassees' perspectives.* Manuscript submitted for publication.

Sharkey, W. F., & Stafford, L. (1990). Responses to embarrassment. *Human Communication Research, 17,* 315–342.

Sharkey, W. F., & Waldron, V. R. (1990, November). *Subordinates' perception of intentional embarrassment in the work place.* Paper presented at the meeting of the Speech Communication Association, Chicago.

Shaver, P., Schwartz, J., Kirson, D., & O'Connor, C. (1987). Emotional knowledge: Further exploration of a prototype approach. *Journal of Personality and Social Psychology, 52,* 1061–1086.

Shearn, D., Bergman, E., Hill, K., Abel, A., & Hinds, L. (1990). Facial coloration and temperature responses in blushing. *Psychophysiology, 27,* 687–693.

Shearn, D., Bergman, E., Hill, K., Abel, A., & Hinds, L. (1992). Blushing as a function of audience size. *Psychophysiology, 29,* 431–436.

Sherman, S. J. (1980). On the self-erasing nature of errors of prediction. *Journal of Personality and Social Psychology, 39,* 211–221.

Shields, S. A., Mallory, M. E., & Simon, A. (1990). The experience and symptoms of blushing as a function of age and reported frequency of blushing. *Journal of Nonverbal Behavior, 14,* 171–187.

Shimanoff, S. B. (1984). Commonly named emotions in everyday conversations. *Perceptual and Motor Skills, 58,* 514.

Shott, S. (1979). Emotion and social life: A symbolic interactionist analysis. *American Journal of Sociology, 84,* 1317–1334.

Silver, M., Sabini, J., & Parrott, W. G. (1987). Embarrassment: A dramaturgic account. *Journal for the Theory of Social Behavior, 17,* 47–61.

Simon, A., & Shields, S. A. (1996). Does complexion color affect the experience of blushing? *Journal of Social Behavior and Personality, 11,* 177–188.

Singelis, T. M., & Sharkey, W. F. (1995). Culture, self-construal, and embarrassability. *Journal of Cross-Cultural Psychology, 26,* 622–644.

Spitzberg, B. H., & Cupach, W. R. (1989). *Handbook of interpersonal competence research.* New York: Springer-Verlag.

Stapley, J. C., & Haviland, J. M. (1989). Beyond depression: Gender differences in normal adolescents' emotional experiences. *Sex Roles, 20,* 295–308.

Stattin, H., Magnusson, D., Olah, A., Kassin, H., & Reddy, N. Y. (1991). Perception of threatening consequences of anxiety-provoking situations. *Anxiety Research, 4,* 141–166.

Stipek, D., Gralinski, H., & Kopp, C. (1990). Self-concept development in the toddler years. *Developmental Psychology, 26,* 972–977.

Stonehouse, C. M., & Miller, R. S. (1994, July). *Embarrassing circumstances, week by week.* Paper presented at the meeting of the American Psychological Society, Washington, DC.

Strack, F., Martin, L. L., & Stepper, S. (1988). Inhibiting and facilitating conditions of the human smile: A nonobtrusive test of the facial feedback hypothesis. *Journal of Personality and Social Psychology, 54,* 768–777.

Sueda, K., & Wiseman, R. L. (1992). Embarrassment remediation in Japan and the United States. *International Journal of Intercultural Relations, 16,* 159–173.

Tangney, J. P. (1990). Assessing individual differences in proneness to shame and guilt: Development of the Self-Conscious Affect and Attribution Inventory. *Journal of Personality and Social Psychology, 59,* 102–111.

Tangney, J. P. (1991). Moral affect: The good, the bad, and the ugly. *Journal of Personality and Social Psychology, 61,* 598–607.

Tangney, J. P. (1995). Shame and guilt in interpersonal relationships. In J. P. Tangney & K. W. Fischer (Eds.), *Self-conscious emotions: The psychology of shame, guilt, embarrassment, and pride* (pp. 114–139). New York: Guilford Press.

Tangney, J. P., Burggraf, S. A., & Wagner, P. E. (1995). Shame-proneness, guilt-proneness, and psychological symptoms. In J. P. Tangney & K. W. Fischer (Eds.), *Self-conscious emotions: The psychology of shame, guilt, embarrassment, and pride* (pp. 343–367). New York: Guilford Press.

Tangney, J. P., & Fischer, K. W. (Eds.). (1995). *Self-conscious emotions: The psychology of shame, guilt, embarrassment, and pride.* New York: Guilford Press.

Tangney, J. P., Miller, R. S., Flicker, L., & Barlow, D. H. (1996). Are shame, guilt, and embarrassment distinct emotions? *Journal of Personality and Social Psychology, 70,* 1256–1264.

Tangney, J. P., Wagner, P., & Gramzow, R., Jr. (1992). Proneness to shame, proneness to guilt, and psychopathology. *Journal of Abnormal Psychology, 103,* 469–478.

Taylor, G. (1985). *Pride, shame, and guilt: Emotions of self assessment.* Oxford, England: Clarendon Press.

Taylor, S. E., & Brown, J. D. (1988). Illusion and well-being: A social psychological perspective on mental health. *Psychological Bulletin, 103,* 193–210.

Tennen, H., & Affleck, G. (1991). Paradox-based treatments. In C. R. Snyder & D. R. Forsyth (Eds.), *Handbook of social and clinical psychology* (pp. 624–643). New York: Pergamon Press.

Thoits, P. A. (1990). Emotional deviance: Research agendas. In T. D. Kemper (Ed.), *Research agendas in the sociology of emotions* (pp. 180–203). Albany: State University of New York Press.

Thomas, D. L., & Diener, E. (1990). Memory accuracy in the recall of emotions. *Journal of Personality and Social Psychology, 59,* 291–297.

Thompson, S. K. (1975). Gender labels and early sex-role development. *Child Development, 46,* 339–347.

Timms, M. W. H. (1980). Treatment of chronic blushing through paradoxical intention. *Behavioral Psychotherapy, 8*, 59–61.

Tomkins, S. S. (1962). *Affect, imagery, consciousness: Vol. 1. The positive affects.* New York: Springer.

Tomkins, S. S. (1963). *Affect, imagery, consciousness: Vol. 2. The negative affects.* New York: Springer.

Triandis, H. C. (1994). Major cultural syndromes and emotion. In S. Kitayama & H. R. Markus (Eds.), *Emotion and culture: Empirical studies of mutual influence* (pp. 285–306). Washington, DC: American Psychological Association.

Trower, P., Gilbert, P., & Sherling, G. (1990). Social anxiety, evolution, and self-presentation: An interdisciplinary perspective. In H. Leitenberg (Ed.), *Handbook of social and evaluation anxiety* (pp. 11–45). New York: Plenum Press.

Twain, M. (1897). *Following the equator: A journey around the world* (Vol. 1). New York: Harper and Brothers.

van der Molen, H. T. (1990). A definition of shyness and its implications for clinical practice. In W. R. Crozier (Ed.), *Shyness and embarrassment: Perspectives from social psychology* (pp. 255–285). Cambridge, England: Cambridge University Press.

Van Hooff, J. A. R. A. M. (1972). A comparative approach to the phylogeny of laughter and smiling. In R. A. Hinde (Ed.), *Non-verbal communication* (pp. 209–241). Cambridge, England: Cambridge University Press.

Walen, S. R., DiGiuseppe, R., & Dryden, W. (1992). *A practitioner's guide to rational–emotive therapy* (2nd ed.). New York: Oxford University Press.

Waterman, A. S. (1982). Identity development from adolescence to adulthood: An extension of theory and a review of research. *Developmental Psychology, 18*, 341–358.

Weinberg, M. S. (1968). Embarrassment: Its variable and invariable aspects. *Social Forces, 46*, 382–388.

Weiner, B. (1993). Excuses in everyday interaction. In M. L. McLaughlin, M. J. Cody, & S. J. Read (Eds.), *Explaining one's self to others: Reason-giving in a social context* (pp. 131–146). Hillsdale, NJ: Erlbaum.

Weiner, M. (1992). Treating the older adult: A diverse population. *Psychoanalysis and Psychotherapy, 10*, 66–76.

Welsh, D. K. (1978). Hypnotic control of blushing: A case study. *American Journal of Clinical Hypnosis, 20*, 213–216.

Wenzlaff, R. M., Wegner, D. M., & Klein, S. B. (1991). The role of thought suppression in the bonding of thought and mood. *Journal of Personality and Social Psychology, 60*, 500–508.

Wilkin, J. K. (1988). Why is flushing limited to a mostly facial cutaneous distribution? *Journal of the American Academy of Dermatology, 19*, 309–313.

Wlazlo, Z., Schroeder-Hartwig, K., Hand, I., Kaiser, G., & Munchau, N. (1990). Exposure *in vivo* vs. social skills training for social phobia: Long-term outcome and differential effects. *Behaviour Research and Therapy, 28*, 181–193.

Zajonc, R. B., Murphy, S. T., & McIntosh, D. N. (1993). Brain temperature and subjective emotional experience. In M. Lewis & J. M. Haviland (Eds.), *Handbook of emotions* (pp. 209–220). New York: Guilford Press.

Zajonc, R. B., Murphy, S. T., & Inglehart, M. (1989). Feeling and facial efference: Implications of the vascular theory of emotion. *Psychological Review, 96,* 395–416.

Zanna, M. P., & Pack, S. J. (1975). On the self-fulfilling nature of apparent sex differences in behavior. *Journal of Experimental Social Psychology, 11,* 583–591.

# Index

~